Eating for Meaning Workbook

Dr. Millie Lytle, ND, MPH, CNS

ISBN-13: 978-1502317605

ISBN-10: 1502317605

DEDICATION

To the long line of women in my family who know how to cook, eat and endure starting with my most immediate Mom, Grammie, Della and Meda. I love you.

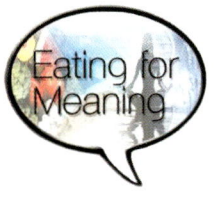

DEAR READER,

Thank you for selecting this workbook. I wrote it as a part of a year-long Eating for Meaning Program. It's a tool to help you understand your own individual nutrition needs. We all want to eat healthy but it can be difficult to stick to a program and know which program to stick to. I am so happy to have a chance to reach you with this workbook, which will help guide you as you confront your individual relationship with food and nutrition. I hope you get more out of it than you intend and I look forward to working with you over the next year. During this time you will begin to explore your relationship with food in a new light; you will come away with the knowledge to understand your own body's response to food and the ability to change.

Please write in this book in order to allow the supplement plan and nutrition exercises keep you on track. Doing the exercises will remind you what to eat and take your supplements. If you are looking for more tools, here are some resources that can help you.

1) http://milliesays.com/eating-for-meaning/ If you haven't done so already, please fill out the confidential health questionnaire so I can participate in your individual health journey.
2) Sign up to get a FREE activation code and try out my Face Your Food APP. You will see even faster results in changing your relationship to food.
3) Group calls and Webis! Once you sign up to my mailings you will receive invitations to regular group calls, webinars, podcasts and email tips from yours truly.
4) You can always book an individual session with me, in person, over the phone or over Skype!

If you are looking forward to getting started right away please turn the page to begin,

xox Dr. Millie

Dr. Millennia Ruth Lytle ND, MPH, CNS

www.milliesays.com

CONTENTS

INTRODUCTION:

> This Eating for Meaning Workbook can help you!

- ❖ Transform your relationship to food.

- ❖ Unlock unconscious beliefs about food and your body's metabolism.

- ❖ Solve your health puzzles nutritionally.

- ❖ Reverse chronic disease with food.

- ❖ Make nutritional change at your own pace.

- ❖ Reprogram your nutritional values through guilt-free, self-change exercises.

- ❖ Heal and rebuild your tissues.

- ❖ Transform genetic susceptibility away from chronic illness for you, your children and grandchildren.

- ❖ Reverse the process of aging, which is important because anti-aging is more than vanity.

"Anti-aging is the prevention and reversal of chronic disease.

Beauty is health. Develop beauty from the inside- out."

This workbook is intended to accompany the Eating for Meaning Program. Originally intended to be done in a year, it can be done in as little as 8 weeks. I feel, however that the more slowly the book is done, expanding each exercise to it's fullest, the more permanent the results. The exercises move chronologically throughout the year in keeping with the 4 principles of Eating for Meaning. Some students may wish to skip ahead, since all principles can be worked on, however it is recommended to follow the pace of the workbook to slowly allow change to occur to you, as you are actively working on the individual exercises. You will get more out of each section if you follow along with the program. Also these exercises are the practical component of the Eating for Meaning, and the nutritional teaching component is not included. These will be accessed from the coaching sessions. You will get more from this workbook than the effort you put in, however you will only get the benefits of it ONCE you put the work in.

Eating for Meaning can help you

(Retrain your instincts, forgive your willpower)

Eating for Meaning is my second attempt at developing diet. Several years ago also developed the Food for Mood Diet. We are all bombarded with too much nutritional information, we don't know which way to turn and the food manufacturers, government agencies and even medical establishment are not helping you! They are hurting your chances of eating healthy. So it's important to take back control. I see food as medicine. If it's not medicine, it may be your poison. This is within your power to change. Are you healing yourself or making yourself sick…with food. You are what you eat and what you eat is the result of many factors (and you may not be to blame!):

1. Personal choice, willpower, craving cycles and habit

2. Training from upbringing and family

3. Availability of food

5. Education (Knowledge of what to eat via marketing, reading labels versus ingredients, peers, role models)

6. Previous or current illnesses that dictate you follow a certain diet

7. The segregation of the medicine from food and nutrition (doctors and nurses don't learn nutrition in college therefore they don't know what to recommend)

8. The deceitful manufacturing of food products ("Big Food" is just like "Big Pharma", a conglomerate that swindles the American public through faulty advertising and cheap manufacturing)

9. The financial gain of government and corporations that control the manufacturing, regulation standards and marketing of foods e.g. GRAS regulations are biased for instance natural Stevia is not Generally Recognized As Safe but for some reason it's active chemical ingredient called rebaudioside (Truvia), who's rights are owned by dirty food conglomerate, Cargill is GRAS. Just a

potent example of how industry influences supposed "safety". The misleading propaganda that GMOs are safe. They are not.

10. The financial kickbacks that grocery stores and supermarket chains receive for carrying "big food".

11. The over-availability of junk food and fast food compared to whole food

12. Mainstream and corporate farming practices that introduce genetic-modification of food and rampant herbicide use and foreign substances into the food supply, without labeling.

How I developed this approach to nutrition

I'm a Naturopathic Doctor and Certified Nutrition Specialist with a passion for solving health puzzles. I put together pieces of the puzzle from public health, sociology, psychology, nutritional biochemistry, epigenetics and of course, nutrition. Most people have been eating the wrong foods for them, unknowingly. Over the last 10-20 years nutrition has taken off in the media and presented us with fad diet after quick fix. We are all bombarded with nutritional information. So much so, that we forget common sense. With all my education, I have to admit that it all started when I was a child. My approach is in part the result of my fortune having been raised on whole food (this is before the super-market chain took advantage of a well-intentioned concept). As a child I somehow felt I was healthier than my friends even though I used to complain to my parents about the steady diet of veggies from the garden, all-natural peanut butter, dense home-made and lentils and rice.

As I became an adult, in college, living and cooking for myself I began to understand and appreciate my whole foods background and instinct for healthy eating. I experimented with this knowledge and different trendy diets. I have been there too! Remember the low-fat fad? At 20 years old I gained weight by cutting fat and subsequently increasing my sugar cravings! Then I chose bulimia as a way to cope with my increasing carb cravings and weight gain. I knew I was on a downward spiral and had to stop. So I started eating fat again and thankfully my brain realized what was happening. These personal experiences provided me with more knowledge than anyone I see on TV. So I made it official.

For 12 years, I trained in Naturopathic Medicine, Clinical and Therapeutic Nutrition, Hypnosis, Mindfulness, Cognitive Behavioral Therapy, Psychodynamic psychotherapy and public health. I blogged about food as medicine and natural health and subsequently I taught thousands of people along the way. When I moved to New York I started mixing all my knowledge together as I became a radio host. Then I got my certified Nutrition Specialist and I brought mindfulness and hypnosis back into my practice merging it with nutrition. I used my patients and friends as guinea pigs ☺ for Eating for Meaning and of course, I practiced it on myself.

This is the result! I hope you will find this information and the process from A to B, or in this case, 1-18 inspiring and satisfying. You will unlock your unconscious about your relationship to food and your metabolism. I am so happy you, dear reader, have decided to join me on this meaningful adventure.

Are you training your body towards chronic disease or are you giving it the most important medicine of all? You can't be doing both. The primary role of food is to nourish our bodies. It fills us, it satisfies us; it romances and seduces us. It gives us energy to keep going, it balances our metabolic functions; brain chemistry, blood sugar, cholesterol, metabolism. Food does this!

Eating for Meaning is as important as remembering your N.A.M.E. because food is Medicine;

We take it 1-6 times per day. It is essential. If we don't take it, we die. If we don't take the right kind, we are sick.

Answer these questions to see if Eating for Meaning is right for you:

1. Are you bombarded by nutritional information and confused about what diet is 'right' for you?
2. Do you believe that food and lifestyle are key, but still nothing is working?
3. Is your willpower keeping you from being healthy?
4. Are you unable to utilize all the nutrition knowledge you have due to mental barriers and bad habits?
5. Do you want to take supplements but unsure if they are actually helping you?

Throughout this workbook, you will receive self-directed nutrition information straight to your subconscious. Increase your own nutritional awareness by changing the answers to the questions. Eating for Meaning is designed to help you achieve personal goals by learning about yourself, because YOU matter MOST!

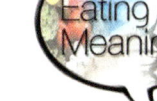

How Eating for Meaning can help you:

- Heal your relationship to food.

- Identify the meaning of your body's symptoms.

- Unlock unconscious beliefs about food and your body's metabolism.

- Give yourself a year to make nutritional change at your own pace.

- Increase joy of cooking and eating.

- Reprogram your nutritional values through guilt-free self-exploration exercises.

- Transform genetic susceptibility away from chronic illness for yourself, your children and grandchildren.

- Increase your own free-will.

- Reverse the signs of aging, because anti-aging is not just vanity, it is the prevention and treatment of chronic disease.

Follow the twelve month workbook while you change your eating habits and order the Face your Food APP and the EfM supplements for best results. The EfM supplements are individually tailored to address the most common barriers to health. Working together, we will improve your body's health while you correct your eating habits. For more info: www.milliesays.com

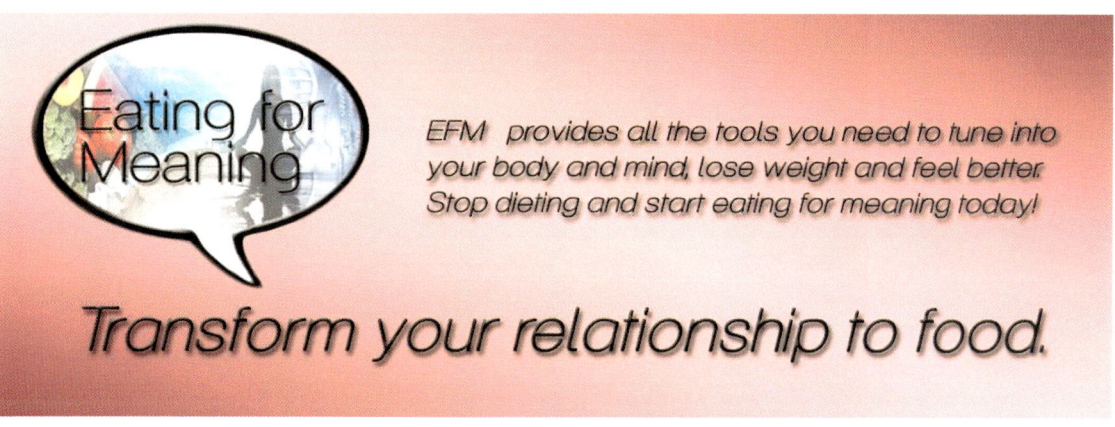

The NAME PRINCIPLE

Nutrition is the most important part of Eating. What does it mean to eat? What does it mean to eat healthy? Do you even have the beginner's manual? Or is your perception of food, perhaps through no fault of your own, so skewed towards fast food and junk food, you don't even know where to start? For instance, do you know that Lean Cuisine is junk food? Do you know what organic food means?

Throughout the course of this workbook I will bring you back to the basics, but not your basics, my basics. The common sense approach to healthy eating.

❖ Nutrition is the most important part of eating- vitamins, minerals and antioxidants, a good balance of fats, proteins and carbohydrates including fiber.
❖ Eating for tradition and community is second
❖ When you eat is just as important as what you eat
❖ You might be sabotaging yourself by focusing too much on taste
❖ Binge eating is a brain biochemistry issue that can be corrected.
❖ Fall in love with yourself not your food.

This workbook allows you to track your eating habits and goals over the course of a year. It offers 18 key exercises to help you understand your relationship to food including; your choices, your cravings and the impact of food on your body.

Once you begin to understand your body's reactions, you can make an informed decision on what foods to eat and when. There are 2 cleanses within the program as well, an elimination diet to uncover food sensitivities and a brown rice diet with option for fasting and mono dieting. Read on to learn more...

Remember, it's important not to judge yourself. You will be looking at yourself from a distance and this is important for learning new skills. But treat yourself as if you were 4 years old. Be kind but firm. You are holding your own hand and entering a new phase of knowing yourself in order to become healthier. This requires patience and understanding.

Last reminder to sign up to **www.milliesays.com** so I can send you a FREE trial of my Face Your Food APP, and more information about which EfM supplements are right for you.

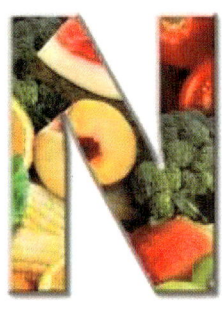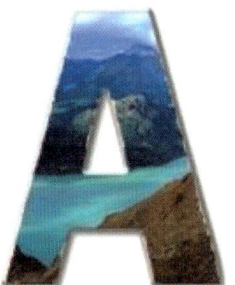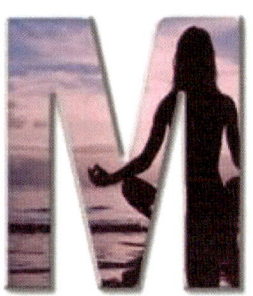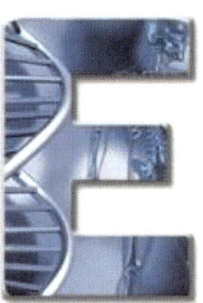

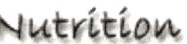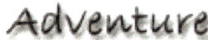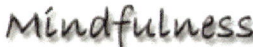

Nutrition   Adventure   Mindfulness   Epigenetics

Here are the 4 Principles of Eating for Meaning that you will follow through the course of this program. I am laying it out up front what you will learn, but over time, you will come to KNOW it for yourself so you want to make the changes from within.

The NAME Principle: Nutrition, Adventure, Mindfulness and Epigenetics

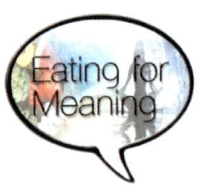

Principle 1 Nutrition N=Nutrition

Ten years ago I debated the role of food in culture with a bunch of culturally savvy artists. My point, and the point I stick to, day in and day out is that NUTRITION, not taste, not comfort, not convenience, not cost, not even our perception of *hunger* is the most important consideration of food. Survival is not even the most important aspect in parts of the world where we have abundance. We suffer from eating high calories and low nutrient diets. Therefore survival is not enough. NUTRITION is the answer. We must eat proteins, carbohydrates, fiber, vitamins, minerals and plant chemicals daily in order to achieve optimal health. Studies show that those who eat 7 servings of vegetables and 2 servings of fruit per day live longer! Studies show that we must eat breakfast and eat regular meals, every 3-4 hours. Food is medicine. Food is energy. If you're not energized after eating you're doing something wrong for you. Nutrition is youth. Eating for meaning, including as much nutrition in each and every meal, will also make you more attractive, more beautiful from the inside-out.

1 NUTRITION = COMFORT FOOD

1 Exercise 1 = 3 DAYDIET RECALL (tip: Don't judge yourself, just list)
Step one to health--Heal the Gut! The digestion is the root of all health. If you're stomach and intestines are not intact, you will generate a lot of information. We need to heal the digestion in order to heal our appetite. There are specific supplements you may be recommended to help building up the lining of your esophagus, stomach and intestines. You may be recommended probiotics as well.
Supplements: (write down the supplements that have been recommended by Dr. Millie and take them at the prescribed time)

When you start using this workbook, grab a pen or pencil and do this first exercise right away. Have fun writing in this book. There are plenty of blank spaces for you to draw, journal and make notes! Start with bedtime snack, evening munchies or dinner if it's easier to remember and move backwards through the day. If it helps, start backwards from the most recent meal or snack.

List all the foods and drinks you had yesterday. Hint: Include number of servings. E.g. 2 cans of soda, 5 cookies, 2 bowls of Cheerios, etc. List all the foods you ate and drank two days ago. List approximate portion size such as 1 cup, ¼ plate, etc.

Foods:	Drinks:

- How's your diet?_____
- Are you drinking your calories? Sugary drinks? Not so healthy smoothies? Sugar-free? Coffees that are more like ice cream than coffee?_____
- Are you eating fresh food?_____
- Do you follow any nutritional philosophy? Do you eat fresh? Local? Organic? Do you even believe in these concepts?_____
- Write a statement about your beliefs about food.

Here is mine:

In selecting food, I try to balance the health benefits, taste and my budget. I believe organic food is generally better for me because it's more nutritious and was grown in soils that have fewer pesticides and herbicides, it also tastes better. Organic and transition meats and dairy have been given fewer hormones and antibiotics and generally the animals are happier. Organic food is generally non-Genetically Modified (non-GMO) and I select it for that reason as well. Although I try to buy organic I know that not all organic is good for me because packaged food is not fresh and still might contain a lot of refined foods and sugar. I prefer local food that is ripened on the vine or even grown in greenhouses to organic food that is raised halfway across the world. This is my concept of balance.

Here is yours:

_____
_____
_____
_____
_____
_____
_____
_____

NOTES:

2 NUTRITION = EAT WHAT'S AVAILABLE

Exercise 2 = What food you buy and have at home determines the mainstay of what you eat

Supplements:

WHAT'S IN YOUR CUPBOARDS AND FRIDGE:

Do you buy brand names or no name brands?_____

Where you get your nutrition information?_____

Do you follow any nutritional gurus?_____who?_____

Do you trust the quality of your food?_____

Open your fridge and List the items you see:

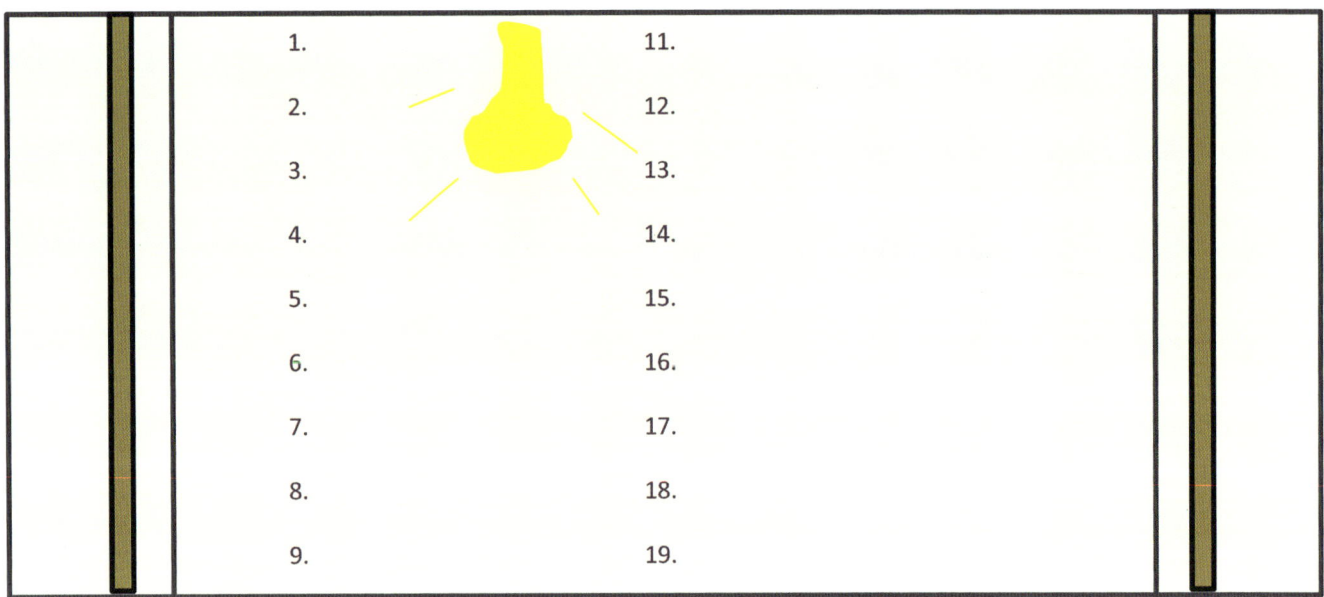

1.	11.
2.	12.
3.	13.
4.	14.
5.	15.
6.	16.
7.	17.
8.	18.
9.	19.

How many items contain more than 4 ingredients?   /20

Real health food only has 1 ingredient. The food itself. Why so many ingredients in my food?

How many items list sugar or four as the top ingredient?   /20

How many items have words you can't pronounce?   /20

Are these chemicals, vitamins or both?

_____

We all rely on condiments and foods with expiry dates to some extent but it's not all created equally. Some of it is healthier than others. Some condiments, boxed foods and even spices have many "filler" ingredients including starch, sweeteners, salts, MSG and chemical additives that can contribute to headaches, allergies and other illness.

Changing up your pantry: "Real food has no labels, so it does not lie and say it's healthy when it really isn't"

Open your cupboards and list the items you see:

1.	11.
2.	12.
3.	13.
4.	14.
5.	15.
6.	16.
7.	17.
8.	18.
9.	19.

How many items list sugar or flour as the top ingredient?   /20

How many items have words you can't pronounce?   /20

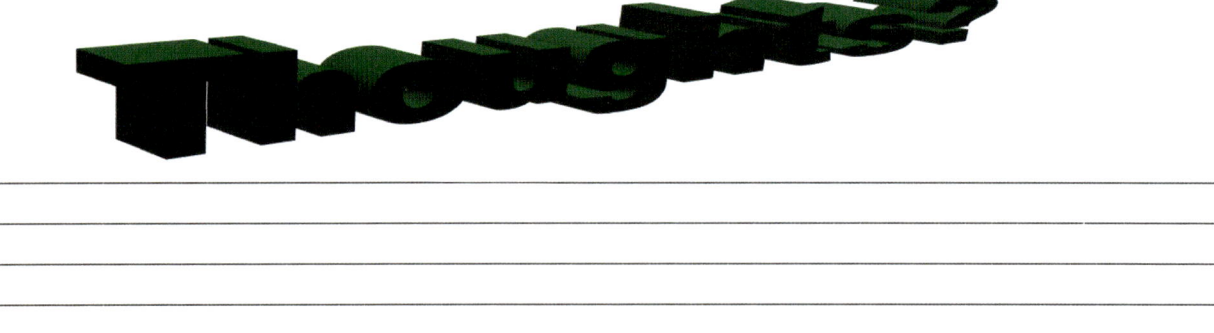

_____

_____

_____

_____

_____

Most people eat restaurant food occasionally and eat at home the rest of the time. If this is you, scan your cupboards and fridge. Notice how much packaged food you have versus whole food

E.g. Whole wheat bread is not a whole food. In fact, flour is not generally a whole food- it is milled, processed and ground, and then mixed with other ingredients such   as yeast, salt and sugar. Read the ingredients, most often white flour or enriched flour often appears in the top few ingredients of whole wheat bread. The food manufacturer markets it as something healthier than it is.

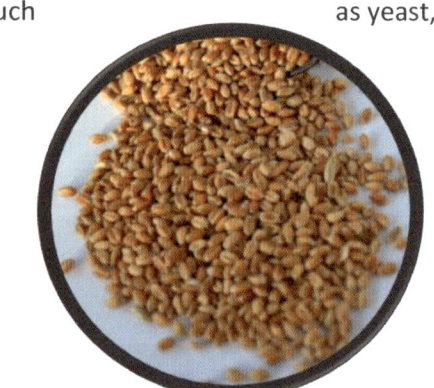

The whole food version of wheat is called a **wheat berry**. Notice how it resembles brown rice. It can also be cooked like brown rice. This is true "whole wheat".

Wheat contains gluten, a protein that causes indigestion or even malabsorption in some people. Rye, barley, spelt, oats, freekeh and kamut all contain gluten. If you suspect a gluten-sensitivity then try some alternatives.

Some gluten-free grains to include in your diet are teff, buckwheat or *millet*

This is millet. It can be used for breakfast cereal, savory or sweet.

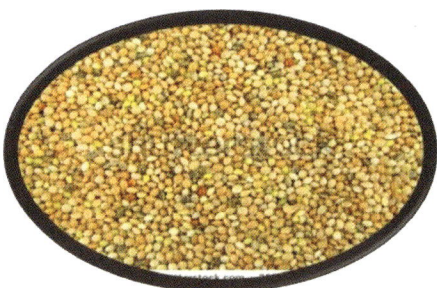

Some seeds, we cook like rice. An example is *quinoa*: it just like you cook rice, even in a rice cooker! Higher in protein than any other grain. Has a nice nutty flavor.

Cook

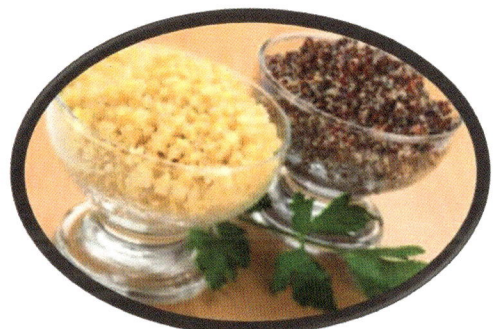

NOTES:

PROGRESS ROADMAP: Here are the 8 Ps of Progress: Fill in your plans and how you're going to accomplish your goals

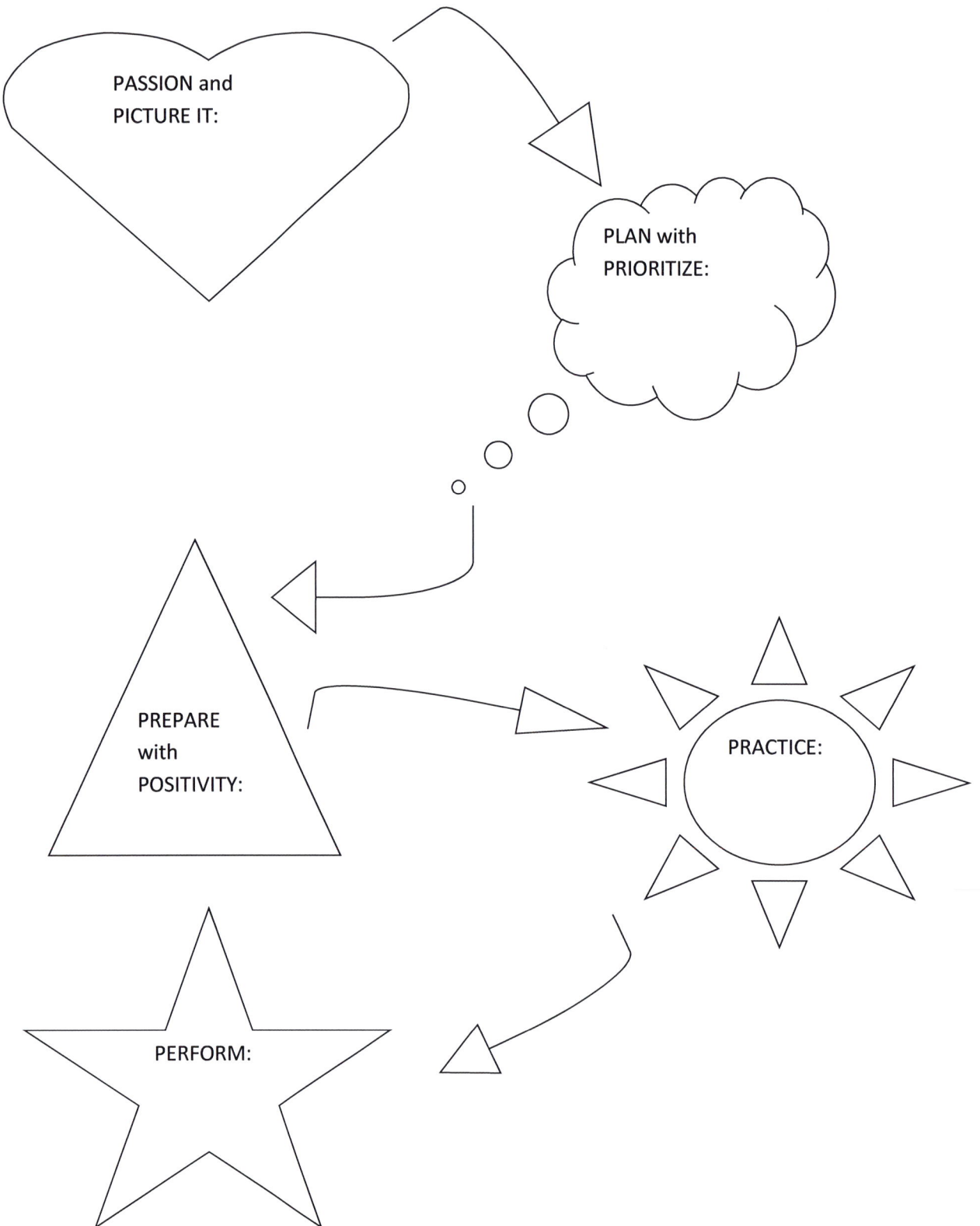

3 NUTRITION = READING INGREDIENTS

Exercise 3 = Know what's IN your food
Supplements:

Do you read the ingredients list?

Nutrition labels or facts panel tell you macronutrients like fat, protein and sugar plus calories but that is really on a part of the picture. Here's the most important part

****

Ingredients: white enriched flour, honey crystals, white flour, enriched whole wheat flour, fructose, partially hydrogenated palm oil, benzodiazepine, crystal meth, yeast, yoga mat, beet juice powder, dextrose, natural color, FC#5, MSG, yeast extract, cochineal

GET THE POINT? IF YOU ARE NOT READING THE LABELS, WHO IS?

In order to tell how healthy your food is, you have to know what's IN it. If you're not making it at home from scratch then the only way to know is to read the ingredients list. Many foods do not contain what you might think. Food manufacturers often try to pretend their food is healthy when it really isn't. For instance, when sugar, white or refined wheat flour, hydrogenated fat or fractionated oils are at the top of the list of ingredients, it means the food is not something you want to eat to become healthy. Or if chemicals are at the top of the list then it means your food is made from chemicals. Get to know what's in your food by looking for hidden sources of bad food such as Sugar, salt, chemical sweeteners. Food Manufacturers sometimes disguise sugar. When looking for sugar on ingredients list it might come in one of these forms: Not all sugars are equal, but it's good to be aware of them

Anhydrous dextrose
Beet extract
Brown sugar

Generally, buy products with only a few ingredients. Don't buy anything with hydrogenated or fractionated oils or sugar in the top 4 ingredients.

Confectioner's powdered sugar	
Cane sugar	Corn syrup solids
Dextrose	Fructose
Glucose	High-fructose corn syrup (HFCS)
Honey or Honey Crystals	Invert sugar
Lactose	Malt syrup
Maltose	Maple syrup
Neosugar (FOS)	Molasses
Nectar (peach, pear, apple, grape)	Pancake syrup
Raw sugar	Sucrose
White granulated sugar	Granulated sugar

So many bad ingredients may surprise you but knowledge IS power. You don't have to eat anything you are not comfortable eating!

Do you use artificial sweeteners like Aspartame? Did you know sweeteners like aspartame are pesticides? They kill your internal microbiome/good bacteria as well.

What if you learned that most of America's farm crops are being grown by a chemical company that makes pesticides (Round Up). Would you trust this chemical company to make healthy and wholesome food?

What other artificial sweeteners do you use?_____

_____

Are they helping you be healthy? YES / NO

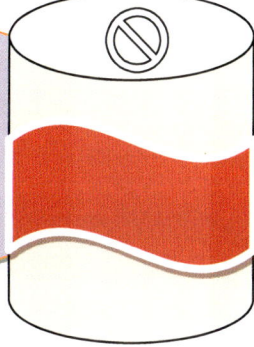

Drinking diet soda is not associated with weight loss or being healthy: In fact, did you know that women and men who drink diet sodas are more likely to drink more of these sodas per week than those who drink regular soda? Drinking any sodas put you at risk for obesity, auto-immune disease, diabetes and osteoporosis.

How many items list sugar, wheat or oil in the top four ingredients?   /20

Substitute this for something that doesn't list sugar in the top 4 ingredients.

_____

How many items have words you can't pronounce?   /20

Also look for nutrients because foods are often fortified with these, have been added back in to the food item. Long names of Vitamins that are often added into foods. For example:

Scientific Name   Common Vitamin Name   Avoid Synthetic Version

Retinol   **Vitamin A**   **Retinol Acetate and Palmitate**

Thiamine   **Vitamin B1**   **Thiamine Mononitrate and Hydrochloride**

Can you tell the difference between chemicals and vitamins? YES / NO

Write down the vitamins and minerals because they can be hard to pronounce too:

_____

_____

_____

_____

Salt: Did you know that not all salt is equal? There are healthy salts and unhealthy salts. Iodized salt, table salt and Kosher salt have only two to three minerals: Sodium, Chloride and Iodine.

Unbleached sea salt, Himalayan salts have over 89 trace minerals. Some of these minerals like calcium, magnesium, manganese, vanadium, potassium, iodine and molybdenum help to prevent high blood pressure and diabetes. The medical world is focused on reducing the quantity of salt in the diet, but the amount of sodium and chloride in the diet are indirectly proportionate to the amount of magnesium and potassium required.

The recommended level of salt recommended by American Heart Association is 2000-2300mg of salt (sodium) per day. If you have high blood pressure you need to reduce it to 1500mg/day. However eating other minerals matters. Other minerals like potassium and magnesium and calcium help keep your blood pressure low.

You need twice as much potassium as sodium in your diet to make sure you don't get high blood pressure. For every 1500-2500 mg of Sodium you must consume 3000-5000mg of Potassium to balance blood pressure and health. An average banana has 422mg of potassium (that's a 12th of what you need). An organic banana may have more if the soil is richer in potassium. You see how it works?

The difference between table salt and sea salt is about 89 trace minerals, some of them essential for lowering blood pressure. Sea salt has them, table salt don't.

-Dr. Millie

Potassium is an essential nutrient used to maintain hydration and electrolyte balance in the body. When you don't eat enough food sources of Potassium or you are on medications that deplete Potassium, you can develop a deficiency. Symptoms of low Potassium or Hypokalemia are fatigue, irritability, and hypertension (increased blood pressure). Unless you have kidney failure and are on dialysis, an overdose of potassium from natural sources is nearly impossible; however, it is possible to consume too much potassium via potassium salts (e.g. Potassium chloride or Potassium sulfates), which can lead to nausea, vomiting, and even a heart attack.

What other sources of potassium do you have in your daily diet?

Source: http://www.healthaliciousness.com

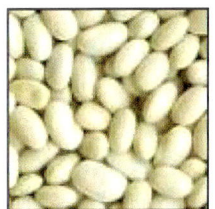

DV stands for Daily Value. The FDA has set a minimum requirement of 3500mg or 3.5g of potassium daily for a 2000 calorie diet. For example, if you eat 4000 calories per day, you would need 2 cups of white beans daily to make up 29% of your potassium intake.

#1: White Beans

Potassium in 100g	1 cup cooked (179g)
561mg (16% DV)	1004mg (29% DV)

Other Beans High in Potassium (%DV per cup): Adzuki (35%), Soy (28%), Lima (28%), Kidney (20%), Great Northern (20%), Pinto (18%) and others at an average of 15% DV per cup cooked.

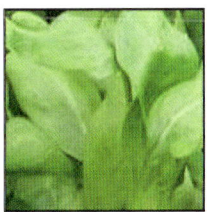

#2: Dark Leafy Greens (Spinach)

Potassium in 100g	1 Cup (30g)	1 Cup Cooked (180g)
558mg (16% DV)	167mg (5% DV)	839mg (24% DV)

Other Greens High in Potassium (%DV per cup cooked): Swiss chard (27% DV), Kale (8% DV), and Collards (6% DV).

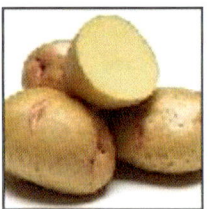

#3: Baked Potatoes (With Skin)

Potassium in 100g	Average Potato (173g)
535mg (15% DV)	926mg (26% DV)

Warning: White baked or fried Potatoes are high in simple carbohydrates and not recommended for people with diabetes. In order to increase the starch resistance of white potatoes, boil them in their skins and let them cool before eating. Sweet potatoes are actually better for regulation blood sugar, though an average baked sweet potato with skin (114g) has less potassium, at 542mg (15% DV) of potassium.

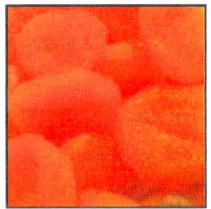

#4: Dried Apricots

Potassium in 100g	1/2 cup (65g)
1162mg (33% DV)	755mg (22% DV)

Other Dried Fruits High in Potassium (%DV per 1/2 cup): Peaches (22% DV), Prunes (20% DV), Raisins (18% DV).
Warning: Dried fruits are high in sugar. The brown ones are organic and preferable to the orange ones that have allergenic sulfates to preserve color. Sulfates can cause food sensitivities.

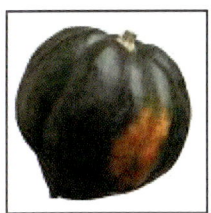

#5: Baked Acorn Squash

Potassium in 100g	1 cup cubed (205g)
437mg (12% DV)	899mg (26% DV)

Other Squash High in Potassium (%DV per cup baked): Hubbard (21%), Butternut (17% DV), Zucchini (14% DV), and Average Winter Squash (10% DV).

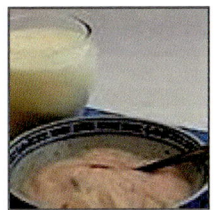

#6: Yogurt (Plain, Low Fat)

Potassium in 100g	1 cup (245g)
255mg (7% DV)	625mg (18% DV)

Other Yogurt High in Potassium (%DV per cup): Whole-Fat (11% DV), Chocolate Yogurt (24% DV because Cocoa has potassium. You can add your own cocoa to yogurt to control the sugar). Although full fat yogurt (naturally low fat anyway) is better for you overall, the potassium is slightly lower.

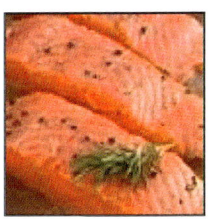

#7: Fish (Salmon)

Potassium in 100g	1 3oz fillet (85g)
628mg (18% DV)	534mg (15% DV)

Other Fish High in Potassium (%DV per 3oz fillet (85g): Pompano (15% DV), Lingcod (14% DV), Halibut (13% DV), Yellowfin Tuna (13% DV), Anchovies (12% DV), Mackerel (10% DV), Herring (10% DV) and most other fish at an average of 10% DV.

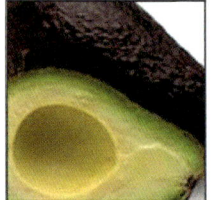

#8: Avocados

Potassium in 100g	Average Avocado (201g)	1/2 Cup Pureed (115g)
485mg (14% DV)	975mg (28% DV)	558mg (16% DV)

An average avocado provides 322 calories, half a cup purred contains 184 calories.

#9: Mushrooms (White)

Potassium in 100g	1 cup sliced (108g)
396mg (11% DV)	428mg (12% DV)

1 cup cooked sliced white mushrooms contain 28 calories.
Other mushrooms high in potassium (%DV per cup sliced): Portabella (9% DV), Brown or Crimini (9% DV), Enoki (7% DV), Shiitake (5% DV), Maitake (4% DV).

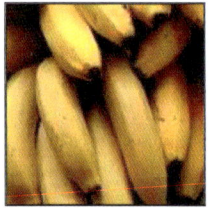

#10: Bananas

Potassium in 100g	Average Banana (118g)	1 Cup Mashed (225g)
358mg (10% DV)	422mg (12% DV)	806mg (23% DV)

An average banana provides 105 calories, 1 cup mashed contains 200 calories

Find some sources of Magnesium in your diet: 1._____ 2._____

Whole food has not been processed in a plant. It does not come in a box, a can. It is not microwave-ready, it hasn't been parboiled and made instantly. It takes time to cook. It tastes better than fast food, junk food and processed food.

A whole food cupboard should look like this (and yes Organic is better)

List what you can change:

1.

2.

3.

4.

5.

6.

7.

8.

9.

10.

Circle the easiest change first.

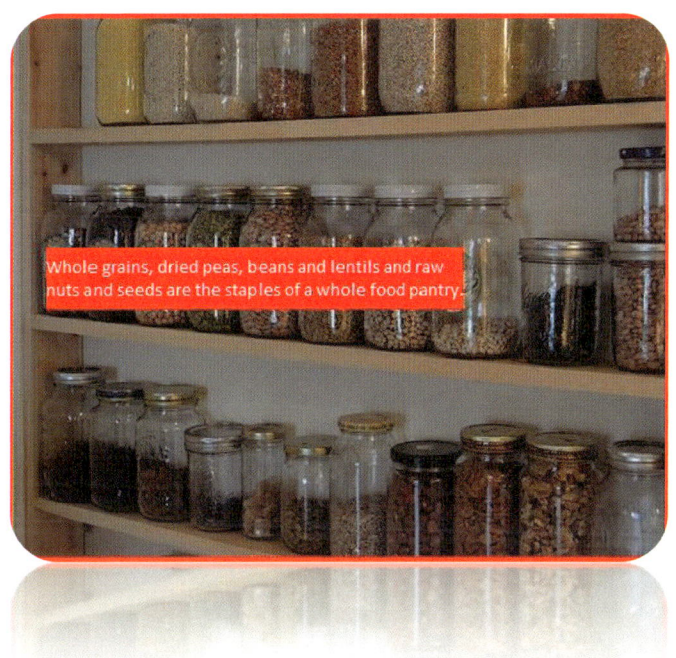

Whole grains, dried peas, beans and lentils and raw nuts and seeds are the staples of a whole food pantry.

Root Vegetable Stew

Root Vegetable Stew: (take 2 days) Day 1, soak 2 cups of dried chickpeas or dried bean soup mix (remember these? shown below) in a bowl of water, enough to cover by 2 inches. Leave 8-12 hours to soften beans for cooking. Day 2: At this stage, extra beans can also be sprouted for a nice crunchy snack and a source of greens in the winter. See sprouting chart in chapter 11)

INGREDIENTS:

Here's a great recipe to get you started! Chock full of veggie protein, fiber, minerals and antioxidant-rich spices.

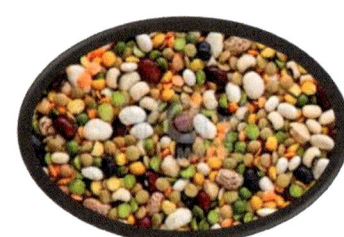

- 1/4 cup olive oil
- 2 medium yellow onions, large
- Sea salt to taste
- 1 1/4 teaspoons ground ginger
- 1 (3-inch) cinnamon stick
- 1/2 teaspoon ground coriander
- 1/4 teaspoon ground cumin
- 1 teaspoon turmeric
- Pinch saffron threads
- ¼ teaspoon grated nutmeg
- 1 pound Yukon Gold potatoes (about 3 large), large dice
- 1 pound carrots (about 4 to 5 medium), peeled and large dice
- 1 pound parsnips (about 4 medium), peeled and large dice
- 3 cups low-sodium chicken or vegetable broth, preferably home-made but carton ok.
- 2 pounds sugar baby pumpkin or butternut squash (about 1 small), peeled, seeded, large dice
- 1 pound sweet potatoes (about 2 medium), peeled and large dice
- 2 cup of drained chickpeas or bean soup (optional and only if you can tolerate them)
- 1/2 cup golden raisins, also known as sultanas
- 1 bunch basil, trimmed and washed (about 4 cups loosely packed)
- 1 1/2 tablespoons cold-pressed apple cider vinegar, plus more as needed

INSTRUCTIONS Heat the oil in a large frying pan over medium heat until shimmering. Add the onions and a pinch of salt and cook over medium heat until translucent, about 4 minutes. Add the ginger, cinnamon, coriander, cumin, cayenne, saffron, and a pinch of pepper and cook until fragrant, about 1 minute. Transfer the mixture to a *slow cooker*, add the potatoes, carrots, parsnips, and broth, season with salt and pepper, and stir to combine. Cover and cook on high for 1 1/2 hours. Add the pumpkin or squash, sweet potatoes, chickpeas, and raisins, season with salt, and stir to combine. Cover and continue to cook on high until a knife easily pierces the vegetables, about 2 hours more, stirring after 1 hour. Add the basil and gently mix (do not overmix). Let sit until wilted. Gently stir in the vinegar, taste, and season with more salt and vinegar as needed.

AND VOILA, NO WORRIES BECAUSE YOU KNOW EVERYTHING THAT'S IN IT!!!!!!!!!!!!!!!!

NOTES:

4 NUTRITION: DIET DIARY

Exercise *4 =* List everything you eat and drink; include the time of day. This week, eat the foods you want every day. It's not necessary to make any changes. Just observe yourself and your eating patterns.

Supplements:

This is how I manage to eat healthy >>>>>>>

I am prepared, even though I rush all the time.

I buy prewashed salad greens so I can always throw a healthy salad together with a little olive oil and lemon juice

I boil organic eggs so I can bring to work

I keep trail mix at home: A mix of raw seeds, almonds, raisins, walnuts and coconut pieces. If I don't have time for breakfast I eat a few handfuls of it so I can stay alert until I can get something bigger before work. Bars have more sugar so I only eat them every once in

I cook a big pot of stew or soup so I can have healthy leftovers anytime.

I carry my water bottle, sometimes with herb tea, bitters or lemon

Meal	Sun	Mon	Tue	Wed	Thu	Fri	Sat
BF							
Snack							
Lunch							
Snack							
Dinner							
Snack							
Drinks							

See any gaps in your diet? You should notice some by now:

1. Skipping meals 2. Eating fast food

3._____ 4._____ 5._____

NOTES:

5 NUTRITION: YOUR OLD FAVES

Supplements:

Meal	Sun	Mon	Tue	Wed	Thu	Fri	Sat
BF							
Snack							
Lunch							
Snack							
Dinner							
Snack							
Drinks							
Feelings							

Do you suspect any foods that might be bad for you? Please list the food or meal and reason why:

_____

_____

SPROUTING –

Sprouts are living food. They contain all the nutrients a food needs to survive life. They are the OPPOSITE of dead processed food.

To increase the nutritional value of your food this winter, consider soaking and sprouting beans, lentils, peas, grains and seeds. Sprouts are a complete protein containing all essential amino acids and nucleic acids. By growing them at home, they are an economical, local and organic green vegetable, available year round. They are high in B vitamins and provide energy. My favorites are sunflower seeds, chick peas (garbanzo), broccoli, radish and barley. TIP: Try making fresh hummus with slightly sprouted chickpeas. Delicious!!! Dr. Millie ND, CNS

Growing your own sprouts is fun and easy if you follow the six rules of sprouting:

- Rinse often (2-3 times/day).

- Keep them moist, not wet.

- Keep them at room temperature.

- Give them air to breathe.

- Don't grow too many in one container.

- Keep them in a dark place (cupboard then fridge once sprouted)

The first step is choosing which seeds to sprout. The standard sprout is the alfalfa sprout. This is the sprout often served on salads and sandwiches and your favorite restaurant or deli. However, there are many other seeds that make excellent sprouts, each with their own flavor and nutritional composition. You can sprout barley, broccoli, buckwheat, cabbage, fenugreek, garbanzo, green peas, lentils, mung beans (found in Chinese food), radishes, red clover, wheat, soy beans, sunflowers and more.

Always use seeds packaged for sprouting (available at health food stores). Buying bulk seeds and grains may seem cheaper than seeds packaged for sprouting, but they may not be worth it. Unless they are packaged as high-germination spouting seeds, only a portion of them will sprout. The ones that do not sprout, will likely ferment and spoil the batch. Using food grade hydrogen peroxide (35%) can reduce the spoilage by killing mold spores often present in bulk foods. Do not use seeds meant for planting. They are often treated with chemical pesticides, fungicides and mercury coatings. Also, do not use seeds that have molds growing on them. Molds produce toxins which can cause food poisoning.

Growing sprouts in a jar

The easiest method is to grow sprouts in a glass canning jar. Any size jar will do. To provide plenty of fresh air, cover the top of the jar with muslin, cheese cloth or nylon mesh screen and secure with a rubber band. You can also buy specially sprouting lids designed for this purpose, available at health food stores or online, etc.

Step One: Soaking For a quart-sized jar, put 1 ½ to 2 tablespoons of small seeds (up to 1 cup if using larger seeds like green peas or garbanzo) in the sprouting jar. Cover top of jar with cloth or sprouting lid and rinse the seeds in warm (not hot) water. I also use a capful (1tsp) of food-grade hydrogen peroxide to wash off any mold). Let soak 5 minutes. Drain and refill so that water is about an inch above the seeds. Let the seeds soak 8-12 hours (overnight as directed below). Protect from light by covering with a dish towel or placing in a cupboard.

Step Two: Rinsing Rinse 2 to 3 times per day for 2 to 3 days. After thoroughly draining the rinse water, lay the jar on its side to spread out the seeds. Do not expose to light. After 2 to 3 days the sprouts should be filling up the jar.

Step Three: Removing Hulls After 2 to 3 days the sprouts will have thrown off their hulls. To remove the hulls, place the sprouts in a bowl and run cool water over them. Most of the hulls will either float to the top or sink to the bottom making them easy to remove. (Note: not all seeds have hulls.)

Step Four:

Harvesting
water and
hulls. Drain in
allow the
Place in an air-
for air
sprouts need
or carotene
(The seed
should tell you
necessary.)

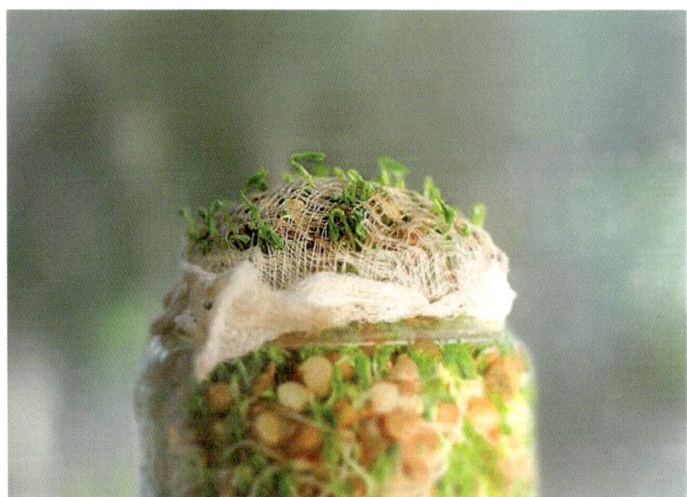

Rinse sprouts in cool
remove any remaining
a colander, but do not
sprouts to dry out.
tight bag leaving room
circulation. If your
to develop chlorophyll
there is one final step.
package directions
whether greening is

Step Five: Greening Once the hulls are removed, place the sprouts back into the sprouting jar or into a clear plastic airtight bag. Put the sprouts in indirect sunlight. It takes about a day for the chlorophyll and carotenes to develop. Once the sprouts are ready rinse, drain, and eat, or refrigerate.

Six: Storing Seeds and dried legumes are easy to store. Put them in a glass jar with an air-tight lid and keep them in a cool, dark storage area. They will keep for a year or more. Sprouts will keep for about a week in the refrigerator if you rinse them once every day or two. Be sure to keep the sprouts from freezing as they are frost sensitive.

FOOD	SOAKING TIME (hours)	SPROUTING TIME (days)
Almonds	8-12	No Sprouting-Pasteurized 3 Days (if truly raw)
Adzuki Beans	8-12	4
Alfalfa		
Amaranth (kalaloo)	8	1-3
Barley	6	2
Black Beans	8-12	3
Brazil Nuts	3	No Sprouting
Broccoli		
Buckwheat	6	2-3
Cabbage		
Cashews	2-4	No Sprouting
Chickpeas/Garbanzo	8	2-3
Fenugreek		
Flaxseeds	½	No Sprouting
Green peas		
Hazelnuts	8-12	No Sprouting
Kamut	7	2-3
Lentils	7	2-3
Macadamias	2	No Sprouting
Millet	5	½ (12 hours)
Mung Beans	8-12	4
Oat Groats	6	2-3
Pecans	6	No Sprouting
Pistachios	8	No Sprouting
Pumpkin Seeds	8	3
Radish Seeds	8-12	3-4
Sesame Seeds	8	2-3
Soy (organic/non-gmo)		
Sunflower Seeds with hulls	8	12-24 hours
Quinoa	4	2-3
Walnuts	4	No Sprouting
Wheat Berries	7	3-4
Wild Rice	9	3-5

I have been making home-made hummus since I was 19 years old. It's one of the first recipes I learned when I was living on my own. Once I discovered how delicious it was using sprouted chickpeas, I have never gone back. People are delighted with this fresh take on a vegetarian classic.

Recipe: Sprouted Chickpea Hummus

Soak 2 cups of dried chickpeas in a bowl of water over night, drain and rinse before using.

Substitution Tips: Add fresh herbs, olives, spices and use different nut butters to change the flavor

INGREDIENTS: In a food processor, blend:

2 cups of soaked chickpeas

2 cloves raw garlic, chopped

3 tablespoons of tahini (sesame butter)

Juice from 1 lemon (approx. 3 tablespoons)

½ teaspoon roasted cumin seeds or powder

Pinch of sea salt

Olive oil (for moisture, as desired)

2 tablespoons chopped, fresh parsley (optional)

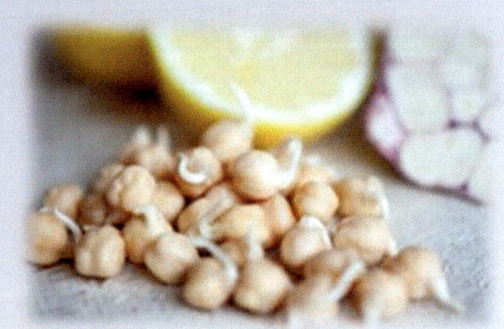

6 NUTRITION: YOUR TYPICAL MEAL

Exercise 6 = Diagram your typical meal including all sides and drinks

Supplements:

LOOKING AT YOUR TYPICAL MEAL:

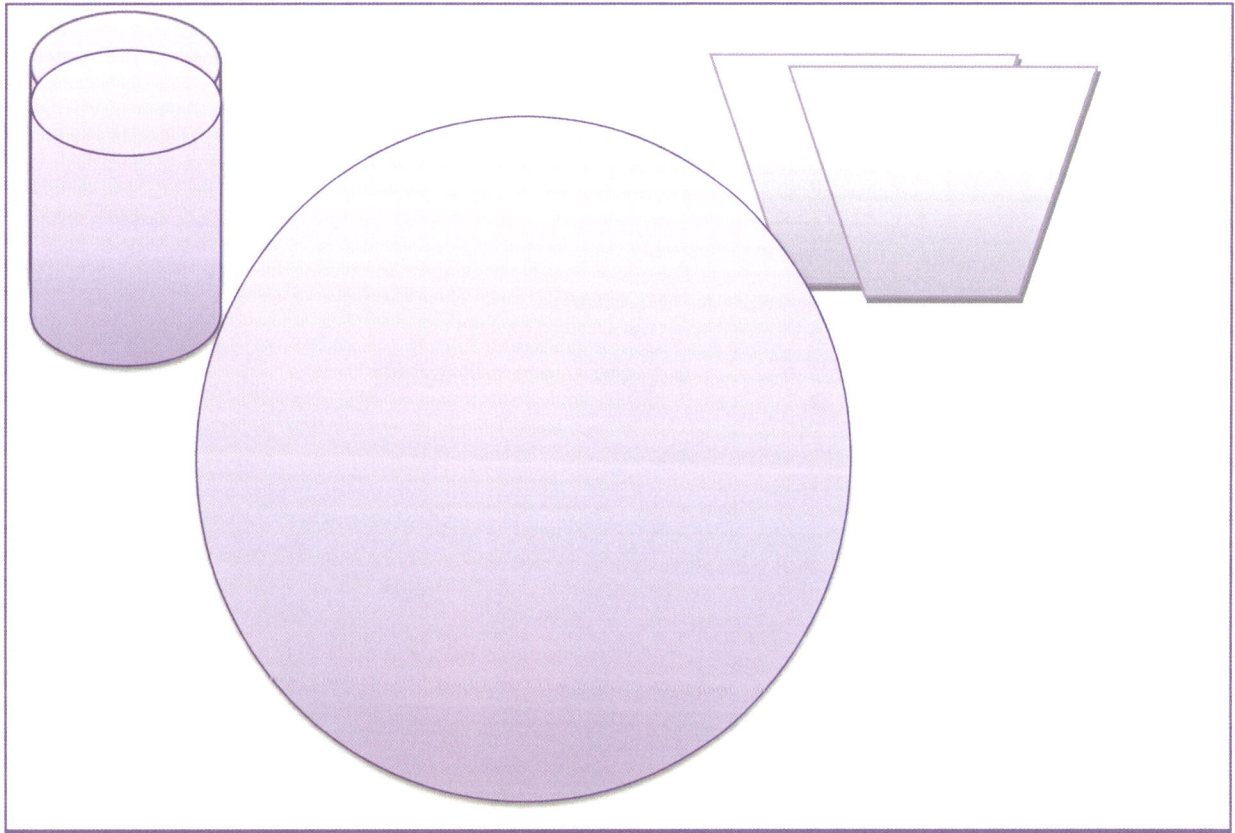

What are your thoughts about your food when you eat?_____

Do you tend to rush through your meals? YES / NO

Do you feel good or bad after you eat? GOOD / BAD Why? _____

Do you drink sweetened beverages? Alcoholic beverages? Milk? Juice?

_____

EATING FOR MEANING WORKBOOK by Dr. Millie

Do you eat second helpings? Third helpings?

_____

Other habits?

_____

Journal Notes: (This is your own space to write or draw your thoughts and feelings about what you've learned so far and where you see yourself)

1.

2.

3.

4.

5. Draw out any light bulb moments, epiphanies, or obstacles in your path.

✖ ➗ ➕ ➖ ＝

NOTES:

45

7 NUTRITION: NUTRIENT DEFICIENCIES

Exercise 7 =
Are you suffering from poor nutrition? Take this vitamin and mineral appraisal
Supplements:

A deficiency of one or some vitamins and minerals is associated with health symptoms. Match up your symptoms to low nutrient levels: Please circle Y for any symptom you are currently experiencing.

ESSENTIAL NUTRIENT

	Vitamin A
Y	Eyes do not adjust to darkness
Y	See poorly in dim light
Y	Eyes are dry and inflamed
Y	Skin is rough, scaly, dry (esp. elbows, knees, buttocks)
Y	Unable to distinguish between yellow and blue
Y	Eyelids 'glue' together, esp. in morning
Y	Loss of sense of smell
Y	Loss of appetite
Y	Skin blemishes and discoloration
Y	Frequent infections of bladder/urinary tract
Y	Dry scalp (flakiness)
Y	Dry nose and throat
Y	Brittle nails
Y	Frequent diarrhea
Y	Loss of hearing
Y	Gallstones

Y	Recurrent sties in eyes
Y	Spontaneous abortion (women only)
Y	Ulcers (gastric, duodenal, colon)
Y	Frequent Allergies (seasonal, asthma, eczema, food)
Y	Frequent canker sores
Y	Subject to constant tension, stress, strain
Total	
	Vitamin B1
Y	Twitching of eye muscles
Y	Puffiness around eye
Y	Frequent blood shot eyes
Y	Fatigue easily, abnormally tired
Y	Loss of appetite
Y	Easily upset or irritable
Y	Loss of strength in lower arms/legs
Y	Pain all over, can't pinpoint area
Y	Tenderness in calf muscles
Y	Confusion and forgetfulness
Y	Gastric distress (indigestion)
Y	Constipation (skipping a day without a bowel movement)
Y	Diastolic blood pressure over 90 (Bottom number)
Y	Irregular heart beat
Y	Enlarged Heart
Y	Delayed/slowed reflexes

Y	Prickling sensation in lower extremities
Total	
	Vitamin B2
Y	Cracks in the corner of the mouth
Y	Red sore tongue
Y	Shiny tongue
Y	Feeling of sand in eyes
Y	Eyes tire easily
Y	Burning or itching of the eyes
Y	Eyes are sensitive to light
Y	Blood shot eyes
Y	Frequent sores on lips
Y	Vaginal itching (women)
Y	Scrotal itching (men)
Y	Swelling of tongue
Y	Muscles cramps in lower legs and feet
Y	'Whiteheads', especially on bridge of nose and under eyelids
Y	Dizzy spells
Y	Oily skin or hair
Y	Excessive watering of the eyes
Y	Have or had cataracts
Y	Lack of stamina or vigor
Y	Unexplained weight loss

Y	Grayish brown pigmentation of the skin, especially face
Total	
	Vitamin B3
Y	Muscular Weakness
Y	General fatigue
Y	Loss of appetite
Y	Frequent indigestion
Y	Red skin around nose and eyes
Y	Bad breath
Y	Frequent canker sores
Y	**Can't fall asleep**
Y	Hands and/or feet go numb
Y	Irritable, easily upset
Y	Hands and/or feet feel hot
Y	Recurring headaches
Y	Subject to constant stress, strain, tension
Y	Depression
Y	Loss of memory
Y	Dry, scaly patches where skin is exposed to sunlight
Y	Burning tongue
Y	Tongue is dark and mouth sore
Y	Chronic skin inflammation (eczema, psoriasis)
Y	Desire alcohol

Total	
	PABA
Y	Have had sulfa therapy
Y	Extremely fatigued
Y	Anemia
Y	Irritability
	Depression
Y	Nervousness
Y	Headaches
Y	Constipation
Y	Early graying of hair
Total	
	Vitamin B5
Y	Subject to constant stress and tension
Y	Chronic headache
Y	Physically feel weak
Y	Abnormally tired
Y	Frequent cold and upper respiratory infections
Y	Sudden dizziness
Y	Physically/mentally overworked
Y	Feel lightheaded when standing up
Y	Loss of feelings in hands and feet

Y	Allergies
Y	Frequent gastric distress (indigestion)
Y	Experience periods of deep depression
Y	Abdominal cramps and pains
Y	Chronic constipation
Y	Low blood sugar (hypoglycemia)
Y	Arthritis
Y	Have attacks of vomiting
Total	

Vitamin C

Y	Anemia
Y	Bleeding or inflamed gums
Y	Easily bruise
Y	Small red or pink spots under the skin
Y	Susceptible to infections, including colds
Y	Shortness of breath
Y	Swollen or painful joints
Y	Frequent nosebleeds
Y	Smoking (cigarettes, cigar, pipe)
Y	Ruptured blood vessels in the eye
Y	Have fleeting joint pain
Y	Known metal poisoning
Y	History of severe burns (including sunburns)

Total	
	Vitamin D (very common)
Y	Irregular heart beat
Y	Poor bone development
Y	Muscular numbness, tingling or spasms
Y	Had rickets (bow legs, knock-knees, bone enlargement)
Y	Tissues are flabby
Y	Dull pains in low back and thighs
Y	A lot of cavities
Y	Deep pains in the leg (bone pain)
Y	Diagnosed with osteomalacia (softening of the bones)
Total	
Total	
	Magnesium (very common)
Y	Poor muscle coordination
Y	Prone to athletic injuries (strained knees)
Y	As a child had partial paralysis for unknown reasons
Y	As a child had failing eyesight
Y	As a child had failing hearing
Y	Myasthenia Gravis or Multiple Sclerosis
Y	Diabetes
Y	Allergies
Y	Dizzy Spells

Y	Bone deformities
Y	Ringing in ears
Y	Menstrual cramps
Y	Crave chocolate before period
Y	Muscle spasms
Total	

Manganese

Y	Gum disease
Y	Physically and mentally fatigued
Y	Breathing feels irregular
Total	

Phosphorus

Y	Swelling in ankles and hands
Y	Occasional rapid heartbeat
Y	Muscles feel weak
Y	Diabetic tendency
Y	Prefer meat to vegetables and starch
Y	Skin of face is more red than white
Total	

Potassium (very common)

Y	Cancer
Y	Family history of cancer
Y	Birth defects

Total	
	Sodium (not common)
Y	Loose skin
Y	Exhausted all of the time
Y	Prefer vegetables and starches to meat
Y	Skin of face is more white than red
Total	
	Zinc (common)
Y	Wounds heal slowly
Y	Loss of sense of smell
Y	Loss of sense of taste
Y	Diabetes
Y	Feel more tired than usual
Y	Acne
Y	Prostate problems
Total	
	Iodine (common)
Y	Feel cold even in warm weather
Y	Low blood pressure
Y	Gain weight easily
Y	Dull pain under shoulder blades
Y	Sluggish metabolism
Y	Dry hair or Brittle nails

Y	Eyes sensitive to bright light
Y	Recurrent sties
Y	High cholesterol
Y	Decreased sexual interest
Y	Dull headaches
Y	Swelling of the eyes, hands and feet
Y	Goiter
Y	Alternating fast and slow pulse
Total	
	Chloride
Y	Indigestion
Y	Excessive belching or gas
Y	Can't tolerate hot weather
Y	Hyperventilate easily
Y	Nervous without obvious cause
Y	Diabetes
Y	Eat a low salt diet
	Copper (very rare)
Y	Zinc supplementation
Y	Pale skin
Y	Fatigue
Y	Swollen ankles
Y	Hair loss
Y	Diarrhea and/or constipation
Total Score	

Do you have any noticeable nutrient deficiencies?

1.   4.

2.   5.

3.   6.

Can you guess why? (Poor nutrition, medications, illnesses or medical treatments, mineral competition, chemical or heavy metal exposures)_____

_____

If you take dietary supplements currently, do you take any of the supplements you're missing? YES / NO

_____

Do you have food sources of these nutrients in your diet?   YES / NO / DON'T KNOW

Notes:

8 NUTRITION: RELEARNING THE BASICS

Exercise 8 = This is how you build a meal. Each plate should resemble this. Choose organic when possible.

Supplements:

Warm tea or room temperature water

1-2 Oz good fat raw olive oil, red palm avocado, coconut oil, seed butters

1-2 cups clear broth soup or extra green salad

Vegetables: Green, yellow, orange, and red veggies: onions, garlics, fresh herbs, spices, broccoli, cauliflower, Brussels sprouts, fiddleheads, mushrooms, salad greens, collards, peppers, beets, turnips, cabbage, kale, green/string beans, carrots, zucchini, squash, pumpkin, radish, sprouts, etc.

1/4 Plate Starch	¼ plate Protein
Boiled potato/white yam, plantain	Wild caught fish
Rice, whole grains, quinoa, barley	Organic red meat, poultry
Sprouted or gluten-free bread	Sprouted organic tofu, tempeh, miso
Organic corn, polenta,	raw nuts and seeds

Serving Size Guidelines

Food	Average daily Recommended Servings	Raw	Cooked
Vegetables	7-8	1 cup	½ cup
Fruit	3	1 small ½ large ½ cup ¼ cup dried	¼ cup
Starch	5	15 grams	3 Tablespoons ½ cup of pasta or rice 1 cup of breakfast cereal 1 slice bread
Protein	6	1 tablespoon of nut butter or Nutritional Yeast 1/2 ounce of nuts or seeds.	1 ounce of cooked lean meat, poultry, or fish 1/4 cup cooked beans 1 egg
Fat	3-5	1 oz 1 Tablespoon	

Instead of counting calories, grams of fat or even sugar – put the food you need into your diet.

The hardest foods to get are the vegetables, but they are also the most important, so make sure you always have something fresh at each meal. If you can't do veggies, do fruit.

Second always have protein. Make sure it looks like it came from an animal or from the ground as processed foods and luncheon meats often contain added wheat or starchy filler.

Whether the foods are mixed together in a stew, curry or casserole or separated on your plate, strive for ½ plate of vegetables, ¼ plate of high fiber carbs and ¼ plate of good quality animal or vegetarian protein. On the sides it is essential to have some good fat. Warm or room temperature beverages, unsweetened, are preferable to ice cold drinks. Ice water and sodas slow your digestion and cause gas, stomach pain, burps and bloating.

One-Dish RECIPE

Try this recipe that includes all parts of the plate. (If you are vegetarian, you can easily substitute the animal products for vegetarian products). *This recipe is traditional French and was given to me by a Jamaican patient. I just love it!*

Fish and Spinach Stew (If you don't like fish you can use squid, shrimps, chicken, tempeh or just lentils).

Good news: unlike other larger legumes, lentils don't need soaking.
Substitution ideas: I use toasted sunflower seeds instead of bread crumbs, the original recipe called for. **INGREDIENTS**
1 cup cooked brown or beluga lentils, **4** tablespoons olive oil, **1** cup raw sunflower seeds, unbleached sea salt and ground black pepper, **1** tablespoon minced garlic, **¼** cup Niçoise or oil-cured olives, pitted and chopped, **1** tablespoon capers, chopped, **2 or 3** anchovy fillets, finely chopped, **2** tablespoons tomato paste, **1** pound or 3 bunches fresh spinach (washed), **2** cups fish or vegetable stock, or water, Pinch red chili flakes (optional), **8** ounces cod, roughly

---

PREPARATION: Drain chickpeas. If you used dried, reserve cooking liquid; if they are canned, discard the liquid and rinse the chickpeas. Put 2 tablespoons oil in a large skillet over medium heat. When it's hot, add sunflower seeds; sprinkle with salt and pepper and cook, stirring frequently, until they're toasted, 3 to 5 minutes. Remove from pan. Add the remaining 2 tablespoons oil to the skillet; increase heat to medium-high. When oil is hot, add garlic, olives, capers and anchovies. Cook, stirring occasionally, until fragrant, a minute or two. Add tomato paste and cook, stirring occasionally, until it darkens slightly, 2 to 3 minutes. Start adding spinach a handful at a time; keep stirring until all the spinach fits in the pan and starts to release its water; sprinkle with a little more pepper, then add the stock, chickpeas and red chili flakes if you're using them. Adjust the heat so the mixture bubbles gently but steadily, then stir in the squid and the shrimp. Cook until the seafood is just cooked through, 2 to 3 minutes.

Taste and adjust the seasoning. Divide among bowls, sprinkle with sunflower seeds and serve.

NOTES:

9 NUTRITION: EAT FOR YOUR BRAIN

Exercise 9 = **Pay attention to the other hunger signals**
Supplements:

- Breakfast truly is the most important meal of the day because it sets metabolism and mood for the day, reduces cravings and gives you nutrients when you need it.
- When you eat is as important as what you eat because a stable level of sugar in the blood keeps the brain happy, whereas too much or too low cause mood problems
- Food is something to be enjoyed but not something but not to be gormandized because overeating spikes blood sugar, causes mood problems and fat storage—however many poor lifestyle decisions cause us to overeat, especially in the evening.
- If you have a food addiction – if the food instigates any drug like feelings or binging behaviors or your thoughts are that you "need" it or you can't live without it, then this is a bad food for you and it needs to be eliminated so you can balance your brain connections.

EAT FOR YOUR BRAIN NOT YOUR STOMACH. YOUR BRAIN IS FIRST HUNGRY AND FIRST FULL.

Here are the most important nutrition tips to live by:

Check which one you can easily incorporate: Make the easiest choice first. This is the eating bible. Following these principles will get you where you want to be with your health. Maybe you already follow some of these, GOOD JOB!

It is important to include all macronutrients, the colors of the rainbow and eat regularly. So many of us get bombarded with all the fat diets and quick fixes and we forget the basics. These basics we all should have learned as children. But many of us didn't, others of us have gotten so off track we have to re-learn the common-sense of eating.

Food for Mood Diet: Key Points

☐ Eat breakfast within an hour of waking.

☐ Mitigate stress by eating every 3-4 hours.

☐ Avoid ALL-CARB meals. Buffer starch and sugar with protein and good fats at every meal.

☐ Remember this: fiber is filling; sugar is killing.

☐ Eat vegetables. No matter what else you eat, never skip the veggies.

☐ Start a meal with green tea, soup or salad to initiate digestion and increase satiety signals. The fuller you are, the more satiety signals will be stimulated in brain to stop eating.

☐ Eat protein at every meal and snack. Yes to organic chicken a twice per week, but remember fish 3x per week, small amounts of organic red meat 1-2x per week, and vegetarian protein daily such as: beans, raw nuts and seeds, sprouts, legumes and algae.

☐ Remember fatty fishes and other sources of Omega 3 fatty acids.

☐ Probiotics take precedent. Strains of probiotic help appetite control and mood regulation

Which one is easy?
Check which one you don't see yourself doing anytime soon.

Why?

> **Don't worry if it's not perfect.**
>
> **Perfection is not the goal.**

S a m p l e   s t r a t e g y :

- Whether you are at a restaurant or at home, try to make your plate look like this. Half veggies, ¼ high fiber carb, ¼ protein.
- Include fruits and nuts/seeds between meals.
- Portion control is important. A handful of anyone food is enough.
- Look for organic animals products, grass fed, wild fish, high fiber whole grains, gluten-free pasta and organic sugar-free cereals.
- Remember you are the top of the food chain, which means you are eating everything the animal was injected and everything the plant was sprayed or Genetically Modified with.
- Always eat some fat with vegetables as it helps absorb fat soluble vitamins.
- Drink 8 cups of water or herbal teas. Drink an extra cup of water for every alcoholic and caffeinated drink.
- Pay attention to reducing extra sugar calories, such as from energy drinks, sodas, sweet teas and juices. Sugar-substitutes are also sweet and not recommended.

What can you start now?

Here's a hint: The following are some of the most nutritionally dense foods in the world meaning calorie per calorie they are loaded with more nutrition than other foods. They may have calories and even fat, or cholesterol but certainly ZERO empty calories here:

Anchovies	Apples	Blueberries
Boiled and cooled potatoes with skin		Bran (oat or rice)
Clams and Oysters	Coconut oil	Cranberries
Egg yolks (with the whites, but not whites alone)		
Garlic and onions	Kale	Liver (chicken and calf)
Small Mackerel	Nutritional Yeast	Tea (herbal/green) raw olive oil
Salmon (wild)	Sardines	Seaweed
Wild rice	(nori, hijiki, wakame, arame)	
Seeds	(flax, chia, hemp and pumpkin)	
Quinoa	Wheat germ	

Want to know which foods to eat regularly? These ones are the most nutritionally dense, meaning each of these is PACKED with nutrients that **fill** your **brain**, fill your **stomach** and **reduce food cravings**.

NOTES:

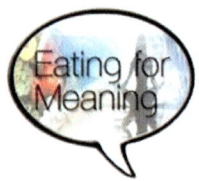

PRINCIPLE 2 ADVENTURE A = Adventure

It's not enough to eat the same 5 foods every day. You must tailor your foods to the season to the location and to the availability. You must mix up your foods to include a large variety. Eating the same foods all the time will give you nutrient deficiencies. If it is indeed possible to acquire all our nutrients from food, it is only through eating a variety of foods that you can accomplish this. Remember we live in a toxic world and acquiring a variety of nutrients helps us combat toxins in the environment. By eating with an adventurous mindset you will enjoy your food more. You will enjoy the preparation of food. You will enjoy the process of shopping for food. And guess what? Your palate, your taste buds and appetite WILL change as well!!

10 ADVENTURE; THE ELIMINATION DIET

Exercise 10 = Get to the bottom of your symptoms
Let the Detox Begin. After the gut is healed then we can detox to liberate the toxins, hormones, heavy metals and drug metabolites your body has been holding onto. These toxins are called 'obesogens' and they promote sluggish metabolism, high cholesterol, high insulin and a fatty liver.
<u>Supplements:</u>

Here we go! This is intense adventure that will crash course you into understanding how your body uses food. Change up your diet for 2 weeks! See how you feel. See how much weight you lose. See how much you learn about yourself! Some foods you may have thought are healthy are common allergens. They might be making you sick. A modified brown rice diet is beneficial as it combines low allergy whole foods with a clean diet, mostly prepared by you. It incorporates the temporary removal of Gluten, dairy, sugar and packaged/canned foods. It prioritizes the removal of alcohol, vinegars and processed foods. You will feel better and lose weight on this diet. Here's how you do it:

GROCERY LIST

Healthy crackers (Annie's, Finn Crisps, Wasa)		Organic Olive Oil	
Organic Apples			
Organic Miso	Buckwheat groats	Coconut water	Dried Chickpeas
Organic unpasteurized sauerkraut		Tempeh	
Raw almonds	Brown or beluga lentils	Brown rice	Apple cider vinegar
Salt Cod fish	Nutritional Yeast (Bob's Red Mill or Lewis Labs)		
Seaweed (nori, dulse, wakame)	Lemons	Flaxseeds	Sweet potatoes
Tahini	Fresh mackerel	Blueberries	Broccoli · Radishes

GUIDELINES

- Organic fruits and vegetables as much as possible. Wash them thoroughly to remove pesticides and contaminants. Use vinegar for washing fruits and vegetables. Rinse well.
- Read all food labels thoroughly to find added ingredients you may need to avoid.
- Avoid specific foods that cause a reaction to you: tingling, itchiness, swelling, smarting, hives, bloating, gas, sensation of fullness, heartburn. You are definitely sensitive to those and you will need to eliminate them for at least 3-12 months.
- allergy-free cookbook

Keep in mind this list could vary in some people. If you find yourself reacting to any "safe" food then eliminate it from the diet.

Vegetables

Foods to Eat	Foods to Avoid
• **All safe fresh vegetables (incorporate onions, garlics, beets, leeks, celery, cauliflower, Brussel sprouts, cabbage, kale, green beans, snow peas, green peas, broccoli, asparagus, fiddle heads, sea asparagus, leafy greens- kale, mustard greens, dandelion, turnip greens, bok choy, spinach, Swiss chard, cucumbers, celery, carrots)** • **Fresh herbs** • **Try sprouting p. 89 esp. in the winter- fresh freshies all yeaer long.** • **Sea vegetables (kelp, kelp noodles, dulse, wakame, arame, nori paper, seaweed salad)**	• Tomatoes, corn, mushrooms (except shitakes), potatoes/potato chips, eggplant, all peppers- sweet and hot and Tabasco or hot pepper sauces/chili sauces, salsa, • canned or jarred vegetables

Can be eaten raw, steamed, boiled, lightly sautéed. Baked is not as good. No frying

Fruits

Foods to Eat	Foods to Avoid
• **dark berries- blueberries, raspberries, cranberries, blackberries, service berries, pears** • **Fruit sauces (pears) with no added sugar** • **Lemons and lemon water** • **Grapefruit**	• Bananas, citrus (oranges) • dried fruits, • kiwi, pineapple, strawberries, melons (cantaloupe, honeydew, watermelon), grapes- red and purple • Fruits that elicit any symptoms

Eat fruit by itself or ½ hour before or 2 hours after a meal, unless using in fruit smoothie

Grains and starchy vegetables

- **Brown rice, millet, buckwheat, quinoa, tapioca, amaranth, teff**
- **Brown rice and other gluten-free pasta and wraps**
- **Gluten-free cereals made from these grains**
- **See Bob's Red Mill grain products or bulk products**
- **Sprouted wheat and Ezekiel bread (read labels)**
- **Yukon gold potatoes, blue potatoes, sweet potatoes**
- **Shirotaki "miracle" noodles**

- All gluten-containing grains (wheat, rye, barley, kamut, spelt, Oats)
- Wheat meat/seitan
- White potatoes (Idaho, red skins)
- Corn, popcorn, corn syrup, corn starch, corn oil
- and all corn products
- Most common food allergies are from the over consumption of grains with gluten—by avoiding
- These foods for a few weeks it gives your body a chance to relax and detoxify.

All starchy vegetables should be boiled, steamed or sautéed, not fried.

Legumes

- **Sprouts (see p. 89)**
- **sprouted organic soy, sprouted**
- **All legumes/beans (adzuki bean, mung, navy bean, black, kidney, pinto, etc.)**
- **Bean pastas – cellophane noodles from mung bean, aduki beans)**
- **Fermented organic soya if safe (unpasteurized miso, Bragg's Amino Sauce, tempeh, wheat free tamari/soy sauce**
- **Peas (all varieties dried/split/fresh)**
- **Lentils (all varieties – brown, green, red, French, beluga)**

- non-organic soy products (soy sauce, TVP, soy nuts, pasteurized miso, edamame)
- Peanuts and peanut butter

Nuts and Seeds

- **cashews, Brazil nuts, hazelnuts, pecans, walnuts as long as they are safe. If you have an allergy to tree nuts-don't go there.**
- **flax seeds, pumpkin seeds, sunflower seeds, chia, hemp**
- **oils and butters made from these**
- **Almond/cashew/pumpkin seed butter**

- peanuts and peanut butter (are really legumes)
- macadamia nuts
- safflower
- sesame seed and tahini
- any nuts that give symptoms

Eat nuts and seeds raw and unsalted. Lightly toast a home in toaster oven or on stove-top.

Animal Products

- **free-range chicken, turkey**
- **organic lamb, beef, wild game**
- **wild cold water fish (salmon, halibut, cod, mackerel, sardines); please note that most canned fish is farmed, check labels**
- **freshwater white fish and trout**
- **rice milk sour cream or tofu sour cream**
- **organic goat yogurt if safe**

- processed meats (luncheon meats, bacon, ham, hotdogs, sausage, canned meats)
- shell-fish, catfish, canned fish
- dairy (milk, cheeses, butter) including brie, camembert, blue, Roquefort, cream cheese
- eggs
- Dairy products are also among the most likely foods to cause allergies

Eat animal protein baked, broiled, poached, streamed or grilled. Opt out of frying and BBQ as it damages their proteins and fats.

Condiments

- **fresh lemon juice, brown rice vinegar, apple cider vinegar with mother/cold pressed not distilled**
- **Celtic sea salt and Himalayan crystal salt,**
- **seaweeds, olive oil, flax seed oil**
- **Fresh herbs: parsley, coriander, mint, basil**
- **Spices(cumin, turmeric, curry, fennel, basil, cinnamon, clove, ginger, schizandra)**
- **Spreads: tahini paste, nut butters, bean dips**
- **Sauces: pesto (no cheese), mustard (no additives)**
- **Brewers or Nutritional Yeast**

- All other vinegars, salad dressings, commercials sauces, soya sauce, teriyaki, tamari- with wheat, pasteurized miso
- Additives: MSG, corn starch, caramel, invert sugar, natural flavors, fructose, dextrose, glucose,
- Refined oils, margarine, shortening
- All sweeteners (corn/rice, brown/white sugar, fancy molasses, etc.)
- Any herbs you might be allergic to: Echinacea, chamomile, lavender

- **Sweeteners: stevia, pure maple syrup, buckwheat honey, blackstrap molasses**
- **Pure bitters – gentian, black seed**

Don't heat flax oil, instead mix into cooked porridge, drizzle over salad/steamed veggies/grains; add to fruit smoothie

Beverages

- **Filtered water, LOTS! 2-3 liters/gallons per day with lemon, cucumber or plain**
- **100% fruit and vegetable juices that are safe**
- **herbal teas: roobois, for example Yogi or Bija or Traditional Medicinal teas, peppermint, licorice, passion flower, milk thistle, Fresh herb teas, dandelion root, chicory root**
- **green tea**
- **rice milk, Eden soy, WestSoy or SoNice soy milk, unsweetened almond milk, coconut milk**
- **Seltzer/soda water (does not replace water)**
- **Unsweetened Kombucha (try the GTs Enlighten Green)**

- coffee
- black tea
- cola and all soda pop/water
- cow dairy and goat dairy
- all fruit drinks high in refined sugars
- all vegetable drinks high in salt (V-8)
- Energy drinks
- club soda/tonic water

Never drink sweetened beverages on a cleanse, not even calorie-free. Focus on unsweetened teas, water and seltzer or fizzy spring water if you want something bubbly.

Reintroduction Phase: Challenge the foods you suspect you are sensitive to. Eat 3 servings of one suspect food in one day. See if your symptoms return. Wait 3 days before introducing another food. This period could last weeks or months, if you are allergic to many foods. If this is the case, you must be taking supplements to your gut

Choose suspect foods first:

1. Cow dairy and milk products
2. Wheat and gluten
3. Tomatoes, potatoes, peppers
4. Corn

5. Eggs
6. Avocado and banana
7. Beer
8. Wine

What did you learn?

_____

_____

_____

_____

_____

How does this change how you will eat?

_____

_____

Which parts of the elimination diet could you keep long term?

_____

_____

_____

NOTES:

11 ADVENTURE: TRAVEL THE WORLD OF FOOD

> **Exercise 11 =** Find good food; what could make you change what and how much you eat?
>
> **Supplements:**

Change factors:

1. More education
2. Stopping Cravings
3. More Time on your hands
4. More organization
5. Better grocery stores
6. Closer grocery stores
7. Cooking skills

What practical steps can you take starting today to make nutrition easier?

a. Shop in advance
b. Cook the day before
c. Avoid fast food- set limits for yourself- do not go to fast food
d. Shop the perimeter of the grocery store (Do not buy treats or junk food for the house)
e. Eat homemade popcorn not chips—making something takes longer so more of a deterrent to eat something bad
f. Prewash and precut fruits and vegetables so they are easy to access or buy pre-washed (more expensive)
g. The palate can change
   a. Just because you love Hagen Daaz double fudge monkey ice cream all day long now, does not mean that is what you will want forever.
   b. The bland foods are beneficial. Foods that are not as tasty deserve more respect. They provide nutrition. Because you don't want them all

day long is a positive thing, because you will only eat enough to feed your brain. Increase bland foods like beans, lentils, vegetables, raw nuts and seeds.

c. By introducing a variety of foods into your diet, you nutrition levels increase and your brain chemistry can change your decisions about what to eat.

What new foods have you introduced since starting this workbook?

1.

2.

3.

What foods have you stopped eating?   How do YOU FEEL?

1.

2.

3.

Do you know where your food comes from?

	Hubby	The barn	
Store/7-11	Mother	The pasture	In my garden
A can	Daughter	Grocery store	Mexico
Restaurant	Son	The pen	Brazil
Homemade	Grandma	The coup	Spain
Microwave	Neighbor	The ocean	USA
A Box	Personal chef	The lake	Canada
Take-out	Delivery service	The fisheries	India
Grocery Delivery	The factory	The hatch	Japan
Fast-Food	Factory Farm	The plant	Taiwan
My own hands	China	The factory	Globally
The freezer	Organic Farm	Monsanto/GMO	Who knows?
Loved one	Biodynamic Farm	Organic farm	
Wife	The ground	Mennonite farm	

There are restaurants that guarantee local, fresh whole foods.

Do you have any in your neighborhood? Make a plan to eat there this month.

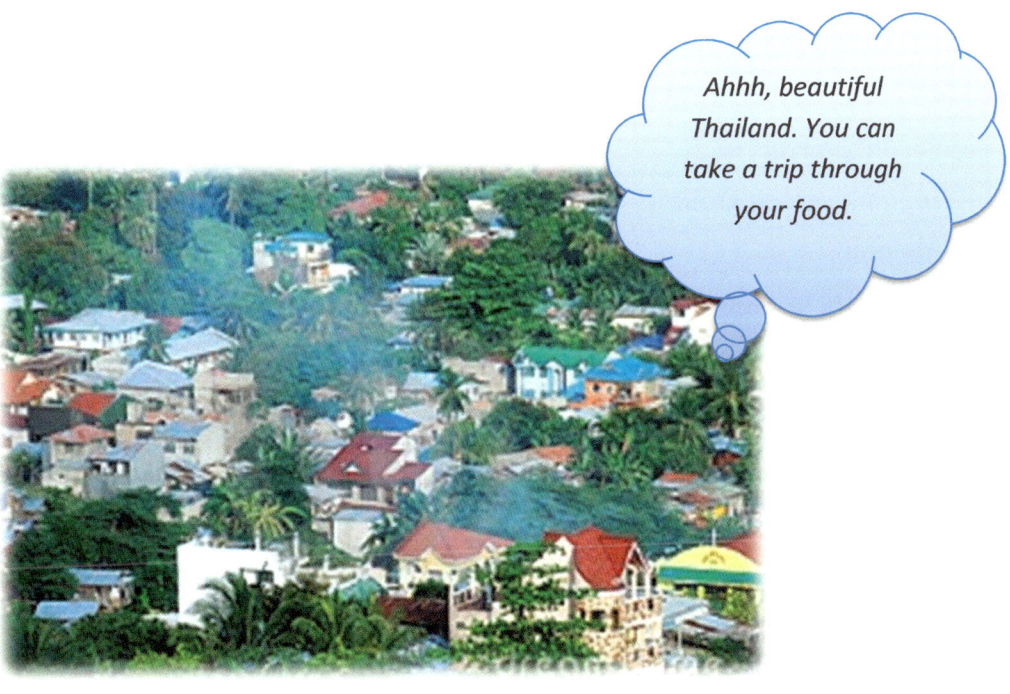

12 ADVENTURE: CHANGE YOUR APPETITE

Exercise 12 = Add variety into your diet
Supplements:

EAT A NEW FOOD:

This month, be adventurous with your shopping. Go to new locations to find your food.

- Farmers markets
- International green grocers
- Health food stores
- Organic aisles of grocery stores
- Community garden or farm share
- Where else can you go to purchase good food?

Exercise: Ask people where to get good food: What did you learn?

_____

Your test this week: Anything you think don't recognize…. try it. Pair it with another food you like, or substitute it for a food you would normally eat.

I.e. substitute edoes for potatoes. of tuber in the taro family. It has value but not as starchy and does inflammation in the joints like do

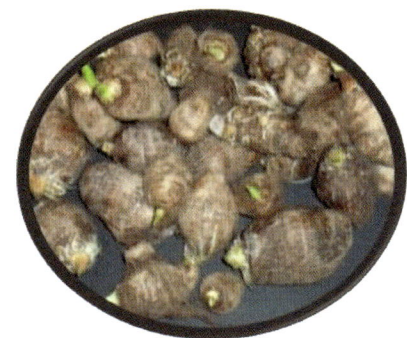

An edo is a type high nutritional not cause white potatoes

Blue potatoes taste like potatoes antioxidants similar to blueberries

but they have in them.

TASK: Add One Food You Don't Recognize Per Week: SELECT YOUR DEGREE OF DIFFICULTY:

EASY: Go to a vegetable store you have never been to. Choose a vegetable or fruit that you do not recognize. Anything you do not know what it is, pick it up, hold it, smell it.

MODERATE: Ask someone what it's called and ask how to prepare it.

DIFFICULT: Bring that food home, cook it and eat it. What degree of difficulty will you choose?   EASY   MODERATE   DIFFICULT

Key points to remember:

Expanding your diet will narrow your waist line. Variety is the result of trying every fruit, vegetable and bean you've never tried. And introducing them into your diet on the regular.

HOW TO GET NEW FOODS IN YOUR DIET; GET'EM IN THERE

1.   Make A List of foods you have already tried

2.

3.

Make a list of new restaurants to try: 1.

2.

3.

What RECIPES will you try?

_____
_____
_____
_____
_____
_____
_____
_____
_____
_____
_____

Make a list of new grocery stores you:

1.   Make a list of new foods you will try

2.   1.

3.   2.

3.

MEDICINE IN YOUR KITCHEN

How to increase the nutritional value of most any food.

Food is the medicine you consume at least three times per day. If your food is not you're medicine it could be poisoning you slowly. Nutrition trends currently include eating Local, Paleo, 100 mile, organic, non-GMO, macrobiotic and whole food diets. Dr. Mark Hyman, author of The Blood Sugar Solution has been quoted as saying "save your life, cook at home". But you have to know what to cook, and equally as important is how to cook. Foods that have been prepared slowly with traditional methods may take some organization but nutritionally speaking it is well worth the effort. Of course, in order to increase the nutritional content of your food you add more fruits and vegetables. You can create even more medicinal value by preparing foods in specific ways to reduce inflammation and enhance digestibility, absorbability and nutrient density. If a crock pot cooking is your idea of slow food, then read on....

6 Ways to Turn Up the Nutritional Heat in Your Kitchen

Soaking

Dried food stuffs can be hard as rocks due to enzyme inhibitors, phytates and dehydrated fibers.

Before you eat or cook dried foodstuff such as beans, nuts, seeds, grains and even flours soak them to enhance digestion and absorbability of nutrients. Especially if you are prone to gas, bloating, indigestion and fatigue after you eat this is a key process for you.

All you need are 4 things: 1) liquid, 2) acidity, 3) warmth and 4) time. In the evening before I got to bed I prepare my breakfast for the following morning I take out a ceramic bowl and add 1 cup of whole organic oats (can use rice, quinoa, teff, millet, wheat berries), 2 tablespoons of whole flax seeds. I cover with water and add 1 teaspoon of fresh lemon juice. Sometimes I cover with buttermilk or whey (the liquid from yogurt) and water. It works either way. I store in a warm place overnight, like the oven or my warm counter top. In the morning, the cereal can be heated on the stove top but is otherwise it's ready to eat. No need to cook.

Sprouting (already covered in last chapter)

If you continue the soaking process you can actually change the nutrient structure of your foods.

Just like in the garden, a dormant seed becomes a living plant with water and sunlight.

This process can happen on your kitchen counter as well. Sprouting changes the proteins of foods into nucleic acids, breaks down the starchy carbs and maximizes the vitamins, minerals and enzymes.

For instance, unlike the cereal grain wheat, sprouted wheat grass has no gluten and is rich in magnesium, vitamin C, B6 and folic acid. After soaking for 8-24 hours, move the objects of your affection to a transparent glass mason jar covered with cheese cloth to keep out the dirt.

Most any non-irradiated seed, lentil, bean, pea or grain can be sprouted with regular rinsing in a mason jar. Depending on the size and density, a tail will start to grow within 24-48 hours. Place in the sunlight and continue rinsing every 8 hours to grow a longer and greener tail.

Salting

You may be surprised to hear a doctor tell you to take salt. This is of course within reason. Some people avoid salt altogether when in actual fact you need up to 1500mcg daily. Low salt makes you sick as well. Instead of bleached and chemically derived table salt, or the abundant artificial salts in canned and fast foods, go for all natural Celtic Sea, kombu strips or Himalayan salt to your cooking as a source of about 89 trace minerals including calcium, magnesium, selenium, boron and silica. The point is, not all salt is the same. Adding salt to fresh vegetables can initiate the pickling process, whereby the food is preserved with salt and over time, wholesome bacteria will grow. Make some quick pickles by sprinkling thinly sliced cucumbers or radishes with a generous handful of salt, some fresh dill and weight them down with a ceramic bowl full of water. After 4-8 hours dump the liquid and serve. *May not be healthy for people with allergies or high blood pressure.*

Saucing

While commercially prepared condiments are filled with sugar, starch and preservatives, a big mistake many people make is avoiding dressing altogether. A simple salad dressing with a tablespoon each of olive oil and lemon juice satisfies hunger and increase nutrient assimilation from your salad, breaking down oxalates and making raw spinach more digestible. What's more, a dipping sauce with a teaspoon each of miso paste, liquid aminos/tamari, maple syrup, fresh lime juice, tahini and a clove of garlic is nutritious and delicious.

Spicing

Herbs and spices are not just for flavor. Spices, like cumin, coriander, fennel, pepper come from nature's most nutritious food: seeds. Like pumpkin and sunflower, spice seeds are packed with anti-inflammatory omega 3 oils, healing zinc and protein. Fresh herbs like cilantro, sage, mint, parsley, rosemary and thyme are meanwhile rich in chlorophyll, B Vitamins, and immune boosting essential oils. Cooking with fresh food is healthier for you, and it is cheaper.

Skyrocket your nutrition while lowering your food budget. Traditional ways of cooking are cost effective because you buy foods in their whole and natural state. A cup of brown rice goes further than a cup of white rice because it's more filling. You can't eat as much. Once you get in the habit of preparing foods days in advance, you find you always have food ready to eat and the next meal is on its way. When you are always in the process of preparing food, you no longer need to rely on convenience food. The need for canned and TV dinners, expensive fast food, Take Out and chips for supper disappears. You have your own production line of health food on rotation.

NOTES:

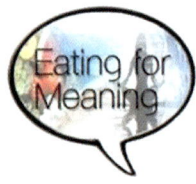

PRINCIPLE 3 MINDFULNESS M = Mindfulness

M: Mindfulness; I always tell my patients to eat for their brain, not their belly. Like I explain in my book "The Food for Mood Diet; Eat for Your Brain and Not Your Stomach, your brain is the first hungry and the first full. By focusing on becoming mentally and physically energized by food you notice how food affects you meal to meal. You also notice how the absence of food (HUNGER) makes you feel. There are other aspects of eating other than taste to focus on. Healthy attributes include the smell, taste, flavors, texture, quality of food, how many times you chew it, and the way it makes you FEEL in your stomach a well as your brain are all equally important. Since we all must eat to live, we might as well get all we can from food, and I don't mean sugar, salt and fat! We must pay attention and act alike a connoisseur. An expert wine maker who is perfecting the senses. This is why it's best to eat at home so that we know what ingredients are going into the food, and also we can adjust it to our own specific palate and nutritional requirements. Restaurants are adjusting the palate of their foods to the masses…and you know what the masses are; UNHEALTHY. That's why you're reading this book.

13 MINDFULNESS: ADDRESS ALL YOUR SENSES

Exercise 13 = **It's not just taste that makes food special, pay attention to the sight, smell, feel, sound and even your intuition when it comes to selecting foods.**

Metabolism: it's time to improve the way your body processes food. By fine tuning your thyroid, adrenal glands, muscle mass and core body temperature, you will improve the way your body processes food. You will lose fat, increase muscle, better sleep and normalize circadian rhythm.

Supplements:

It's not just flavor that's important; texture (crunch, slippery, overly soft, rough, creamy, etc.), food quality, flavor, smell, freshness and how it feels going down are all important aspects of eating. Some people even believe in the 6th sense- intuition. I know I do.

List your 4 favorite Foods

1.

2.

3.

4.

How do you feel about food?

List Other 4 Foods You Eat Most Often

1.

2.

3.

4.

List 4 Foods that are Treats

1.

2.

3.

4.

ARE THESE FOODS THE SAME?   **Yes or No**

Self-Improvement Diary; Are you doing all you can to make changes?

What are your limits to healthy eating?

_____

Why won't you try some foods you don't like?_____

Are you holding onto personal baggage, even from childhood?_____

Do you trust the person who made it to have good intentions for your health?_____

How do you feel looking at this meal? _____

Thinking about eating this meal

One physical feeling: _____

One emotional feeling: _____

One thought about yourself: _____

How do you feel after you've eaten this meal?_____

One thought about yourself: _____

Diagram what you intend your meal to look like. What is your ideal meal?

Do you drink water? _____how many glasses/day__1-2-3-4-5-6-7-8-9-10

Do you eat salad? _____how many cups/day____1-2-3-4-5-6-7-8-9-10

What percentage of your place are vegetables? (Potatoes, plantain, white yams and corn are starch/carbs not vegetables) _____%

How do you feel while you're preparing to eat this meal?_____

One physical feeling: _____One emotional feeling: _____

One thought about yourself:_____

How do you feel after you've eaten this meal?

One physical feeling: _____

One emotional feeling: _____

One thought about yourself:_____

Are you accomplishing your goals?

Mindfulness can also be called 'self-awareness, taking a moment to check in with yourself and your reasons for doing things. It applies to all aspects of life, and is one of the 4 principles of Eating for Meaning. You know you need to eat three to five times per day. Plan ahead. Think the day before what you're going to eat tomorrow. Could you do this? Could you plan your menu for the week, and take steps to eat this way, even if you had to prepare some things in advance? Could you have your family eat with you? Are you eating on the run? Eating in the car? Eating alone? Eating too fast? Eating in the dark? Hiding the evidence? Face your emotions. Face your Food. Face yourself. Even the most minor level of avoidance keeps bad habit repeating themselves. Face the emotion or thoughts that are driving the binge.

NOTES:

14 MINDFULNESS: CHANGE YOUR PALETTE

Exercise 14 = Eat a food you don't like

Supplements:

Do you have aversions to foods you didn't like as a kid? Do you avoid foods "you don't like" because you have a memory of not liking it? What foods don't you like AND have not tried in 5 year or longer? If you haven't tried it how do you know you don't like it?

1.   5.

2.   6.

3.   7.

4.   8.

Your task this week: Anything you think you generally avoid…. try it. Pair it with another food you like, or prepare it a different way than your mother did.

TASKS: DEGREE OF DIFFICULTY: EASY   MODERATE   DIFFICULT

EASY: Go to a vegetable store you have never been to. Choose a vegetable or fruit that you do not recognize. Anything you do not know what it is, pick it up, hold it, smell it.

MODERATE: Look up a recipe using that food that sounds good

DIFFICULT: Cook it and eat it. Use mindfulness principles like paying attention to

How do you feel as you prepare it?_____

How is the smell?_____

What is the texture in your mouth? _____

What is the flavor or taste? (It's ok not to like it but eat some anyway)_____

How it makes you feel afterwards?_____

Expanding your diet will
narrow your waist line

a. Introduce more and more variety into your diet. This will broaden your palate, your nutrient potential and make you healthier in the long run.
b. Variety is NOT a slice of toast for breakfast, a slice of pizza for lunch and a slice of lasagna for dinner.
c. Variety is the result of trying every fruit, vegetable and bean you've never tried. And introducing them into your diet.

Mindfulness Exercise: How would you eat if you were the exact opposite of yourself?

_____

_____

_____

_____

_____

_____

_____

Make a List of up to 5 foods you don't like, that you will try again:

1.

2.

3.

4.

5.

Make a list of foods you generally don't like that you tried this month:

1.

2.

3.

4.

5.

IF you were trying to help your son or daughter lose weight or become healthy, what would you advise them to eat?

_____

_____

_____

_____

_____

15 MINDFULNESS: CHANGE YOUR MIND

Exercise 15 = Change your Mind
Supplements:

MIND CHANGE: **Do you do it or does it happen automatically?**

What do you say to yourself when you're eating? Do you talk down to yourself? Can you make an effort to enjoy eating, make it pleasurable? What would that take to make eating pleasurable? Deeply satisfying? Can you go deeper in your ideas of pleasure? Beyond taste? What's beyond taste? Self-love? Dare yourself.

Now you:_____

_____

_____

_____

_____

_____

_____

_____

Throughout the course of this workbook, you have noticed that food affects your body. You have by now made changes in your pantry, in your choice at restaurants, read labels and no doubt feeling better. These are exercises in mindfulness. But there's more to it: **Food Diary and Emotion Associations**

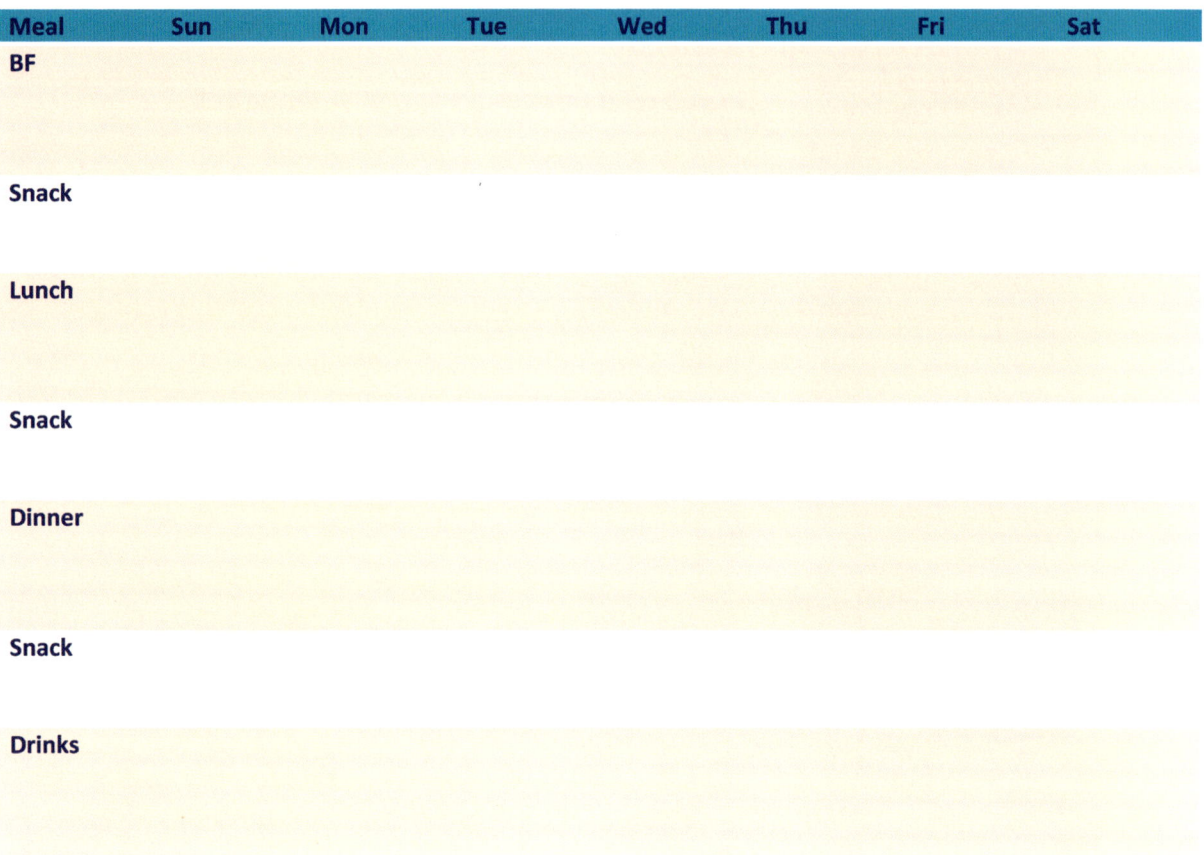

Meal	Sun	Mon	Tue	Wed	Thu	Fri	Sat
BF							
Snack							
Lunch							
Snack							
Dinner							
Snack							
Drinks							

PUT A √ BESIDE YOUR FAVORITE FOODS.

Are there any foods you CANNOT live without? You just LOVE them too much?

1.

2.

3.

4.

Your FAVORITE foods could be problem foods for you, sending drug-like responses to your brain and giving you a dopamine rush instead of healthier satiation.

Let's rate how they do for you really.

Take your favorite foods (one by one). How did you feel after eating it? Rate out of 10, if 10 is the best and 0 is the worst.

- ❖ Energy Level   /10
- ❖ Satiety   /10
- ❖ Mood   /10
- ❖ Texture   /10
- ❖ Smell   /10
- ❖ Feeling in stomach   /10
- ❖ Satiation   /10

Put a √ beside the food you don't normally eat, but enjoy.

- ❖ Energy Level   /10
- ❖ Satiety   /10
- ❖ Mood   /10
- ❖ Texture   /10
- ❖ Smell   /10
- ❖ Feeling in stomach   /10

Put a √ beside the foods you will eat more of.

How do you generally feel after eating?

- ❖ Energy Level   /10
- ❖ Satiety   /10
- ❖ Mood   /10
- ❖ Texture   /10
- ❖ Smell   /10
- ❖ Feeling in stomach   /10

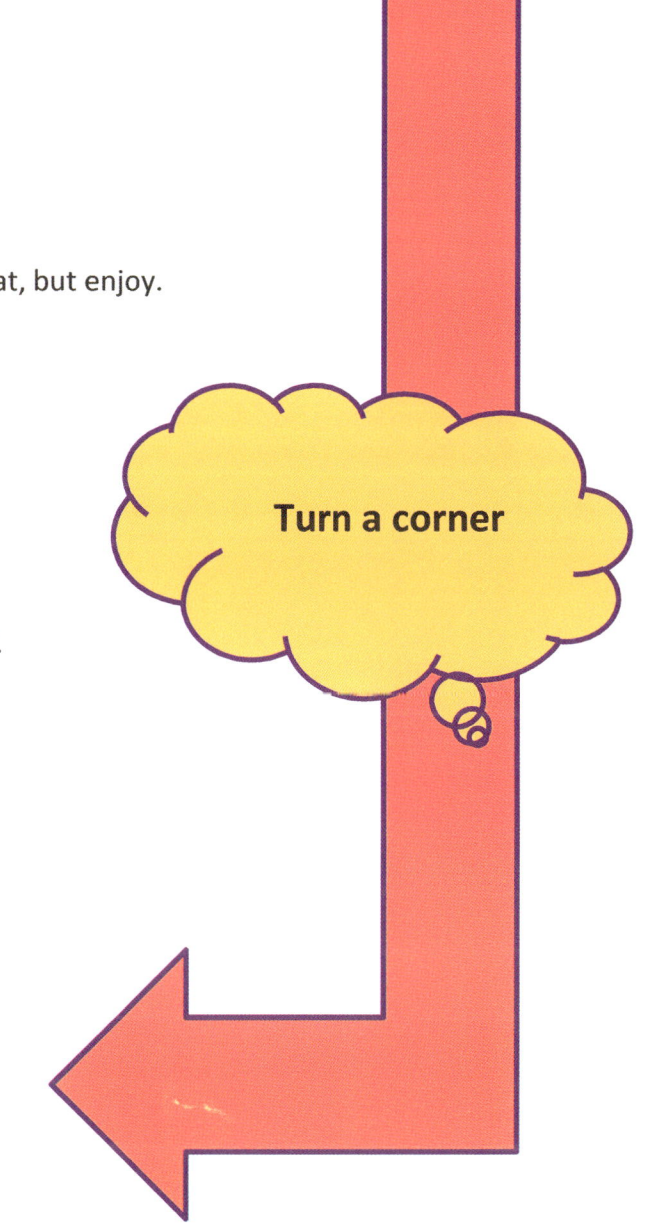

Turn a corner

THIS IS MY IDEA OF AN IDEAL PLATE though it does need a DIPPING SAUCE. Condiments are dangerous territory because so many of them have highly processed sugars, colors and artificial flavoring. Making your own sauces allows you to increase nutritional value of your food in a big way!

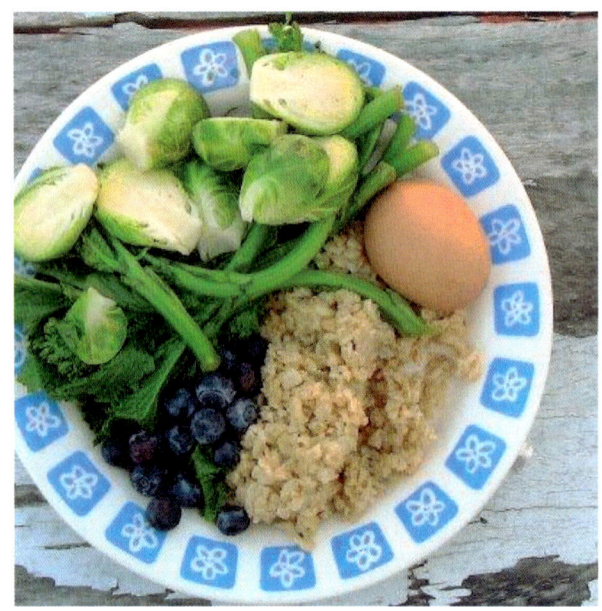

photo credit: Yuula Benivolski

Here is a recipe for my own Peanut Sauce (Can substitute sesame seed or pumpkin seed butter)

In a bowl whisk together: 2 tablespoons hot water

1 teaspoon unpasteurized red or white miso paste.

2 tablespoons crunchy peanut butter (just peanuts- not sugar)

1 tablespoon fresh Lime Juice

1 clove garlic, crushed

1 teaspoon of raw unpasteurized honey

2 Shakes Worchestershire

This recipe adds protein, healthy immune boosters. It's medicine in your meal.

Oh yeah, AND IT ADDS A YUMMY PEANUT FLAVOR

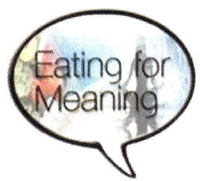

PRINCIPLE 4 EPIGENETICS E = Epigenetics

We are all born with genes. With our genes, in the olden days they used to say our nature. But although we are born with genes that predispose each of us to certain illnesses and health tendencies, these illnesses are not automatic. Hypothetically, just because I am born with a brain cancer gene does not mean I will die from the disease just like my father did. Same goes with people for whom diabetes, heart disease, autoimmune, arthritis and other forms of cancer run in the family. This is because genes are affected by their environment. In fact, a particular can cause a gene to turn on disease or turn it off. Determining what these environmental factors are is the field of Epigenetics. Food, lifestyle, mental outlook, stress levels are all determining factors of your youthful potential. There are numerous studies looking at nutrients, food and caloric restriction to reduce aging and disease. You can even change the genes of you children and grandchildren, for generations to come! Nutrigenomics studies how our genes and DNA are affected by the nutrients we include, or omit, from our diet.

16 EPIGENETICS: CHANGE YOUR GENES

Exercise 16 = **Change Your Environment, Change Your Life, Change Your Genes**
Epigenetics: Even more specific than the field of epigenetics is the field of Nutrigenomics, which looks at the genetic changes that result from the foods we eat.
Supplements:

Emotional baggage is tied along with food- as food is an emotional experienced attached to your identity, sense of self, relationship with parents, self-care and soothing, attachments to the world and people you love.

Has your doctor told you to eat differently but you have no idea what that means?

Why dieting doesn't work: When you reduce calories without a nutritional strategy you lose not only fat, but also muscle, which is your fat burning engine, called metabolism. The more lean muscle mass you have, the more calories you burn at rest. Lean muscle burns more calories than fat. If you currently weight 230 pounds you might require 75 mg of protein per day to ensure you continue to burn 1800 calories at rest. You might be eating 3000 calories and increasingly gaining weight. If you on a diet, reduce your protein intake, and lose 30 pounds you go from burn 1800 calories at rest to 1500 calories per day due to lost muscle mass. You shrunk, you didn't lose fat on that diet. Because you shrunk our muscles you are no longer able to burn those 1800 calories and now burn 1500 calories. The problem is once your diet is over and you go back to eating the same way, you all of a sudden don't have a fat burning engine and you even more weight back very quickly, in fat storage, never increasing your lean muscle mass again.

In order to keep our lean muscle mass we require good quality protein. And resistance exercise. Cardio is not enough. We also need nutrition from specific foods and herbs that allow our genes to switch on toward muscle building. By increasing sugar, bleach, pesticides and other chemicals you are, even unknowingly, causing genetic change that can make you, your children and your grandchildren sick with diabetes, heart disease and some cancers. Whereas eating fish, turmeric, green tea, saffron, and pomegranates can make healthy DNA that keep you young and disease free.

Keep the traditional diet

The foods you were brought up on may be better for you than other foods. Wherever in the world you live, incorporate some of the best of the traditional diet back into your lifestyle. You've heard of "Eat Right for Your Type" but even Dr. D'Adamo has moved on from that overly simplified way of viewing how we should nourish ourselves. His latest rendition is called "Eat Right for Your Genotype".

I.e. in America the Italian diet is heavy in carbs with big servings of pasta and pizza, yet the Mediterranean Diet is one of the healthiest diets in the world. Italian food in America is just not as healthy as Italian food in Italy. In Italy they eat more veggies, raw nuts, seeds, beans, smaller portions with more courses. When they eat pasta, they eat only a small bowl, followed by fish or a small piece of meat and vegetables.

How can you reintroduce foods traditional to your cultural background?

1.

2.

3.

4.

How can you make these traditional foods healthier?

1.

2.

3.

4.

Family Food: Ask your grandmother, your mother or research online how to prepare the traditional version of your favorite comfort food. Rather than the quick way, make it the slow way!

Exercise 17 = Detox with option of fasting
Supplements:

Temporary Diet – as diets are meant to be

This is a temporary diet for the purpose of kick starting metabolism, losing weight, reducing sugar cravings, resetting genes, cutting out sugar, alcohol, stimulants, reducing inflammation and other inflammatory foods like gluten, common allergens, dairy, meat and processed foods.

To succeed at this cleanse. Do groceries prior to the start so you have plenty to eat. This diet is under my guidance. I need to know all your health concerns prior to starting. Foods with highest nutrients in the fewest calories- Under 40 calories per serving (1/2 cup) and jam packed with nutrition: This means you could your weight in these foods per day and never gain a pound!

EFM 14 DAY DETOX WITH 3 DAY FAST (OR MONO DIET)

General Instructions:
        This diet will give you all the nutrition that you will need while your body cleanses and heals itself. You don't have to go hungry, and you don't' have to count calories, weigh food, or pay attention to the selection of food. You eat whenever you are hungry, and as often as you like. While on this diet, you may experience some weight loss. Eat until you feel full, but not engorged. It is better to eat several small meals per day rather than 3 large ones.
Do not drink with your meals, as this dilutes the enzymes in the stomach needed to properly digest the food eaten. Keep about 10 to 15 minutes before or after eating to drink.
Food combining is based on the discovery that certain combinations of foods may be digested with greater ease and efficiency than others. If you have trouble digesting carbohydrates then eat only fruits at one time separate from vegetables and rice. This goes for fruit and vegetable juices as well.

WAKE UP EVERY MORNING AND HAVE 16 OUNCES OF ROOM TEMPERATURE WATER. ADD LEMON OR SCHIZANDRA BERRY.

Arugula   Kale   Garlic

Asparagus   Lemons   Limes

Beets   Boiled Yukon Potatoes Onions

Broccoli Peppers Broth   Pumpkin

Radishes Brussels sprouts Berries (Any Kind)   Carrots

Cabbage   Fennel   Celery

Cauliflower   tea (green and black unsweetened)

Coffee (black)   Cocoa (raw or pure)   Watercress

Lettuce   Grapefruit   Zucchini

FROM DAY 1-14: The Purest Cleanse is Just Brown Rice and veggies:
(As much as you like!)
* ORGANIC BROWN RICE (substitute gluten-free grain or seed like quinoa and chia)
    Rinse the rice first. Bring to a boil 2 to 2 1/4 cups of water per 1 cup of rice.
    After bringing it to a boil, turn to low for **45-60** minutes. Keep pot covered and
    do not stir while cooking. Onions, herbs or spices can be added if desired
    during the last 15-20 minutes of cooking time.

Brown rice porridge, quinoa porridge, chia seed pudding, brown rice congee, sushi,
macrobowls, kitchari are all staples

VEGETABLES (at least half the plate, organic preferably, but may be difficult to find)
    All kinds of whole vegetables can be eaten (except for corn and mushrooms).
    Make sure to wash them very well. They can be eaten raw, steamed or baked.
    Combine them with rice if you wish. No frozen, canned or jarred vegetables
    should be eaten.

Sea vegetables like nori, kombu, arame, wakami, dulse, blue-green algae, spirulina, chlorella
Sprouts! Especially in the wintertime, you can grow fresh veggies at home.

FRUITS (organic preferably, but these are difficult to find)
All kinds of whole fruits can be eaten (except for bananas and dried fruit). Make sure to wash them very well. Eat fruit raw. Eat fruit by itself: *1/2* hour before or 2 hours after a meal.

CONDIMENTS
  Olive/Flax/Coconut oils, red palm oil, grape seed oil, fresh lemon/lime juice,* herbs and spices that contain no salt or MSG, Bragg's apple cider vinegar, unpasteurized miso, tamari or wheat free soy sauce or Bragg's Liquid Aminos
 *Flaxseed oil (this oil must be refrigerated, never heated and used within 3 weeks of opening it)

BEVERAGES
- At least 2 quarts of Filtered distilled or spring water. With lemon or schizandra berries (detox)
- Vegetable and potassium broths
- *Herbal teas, such as detox teas by Yogi or Medicinal Traditional, milk thistle, dandelion leaf and root, licorice root, green tea, blueberry leaf, bilberry, rooibos, organic green tea, etc.
- Pure pomegranate, tart-cherry, cranberry and blueberry juices. *Vegetable and fruit juices – preferably freshly made and organic. However, if they are from jars or cans, make sure they contain nothing other than 100% juice. (Read your labels). Dilute juices with water half and half.
- Green juices – blended or detox juice- cucumber, ginger, lemon, green apple, beets, carrot, avocado, sprouts, Vegetable and fruit juice – preferably cold pressed organic- the best is fresh pressed from a juicer, otherwise juices with no additives, sugar, chemicals, and little or no salt (can be found in health food stores)

To improve digestion, drink liquids 15 minutes on either side of eating.

OTHER INSTRUCTIONS:

See below for protein options. While proteins options are not AS cleansing as brown rice and vegetables alone, if you need some extra energy add some protein options. Restaurant food includes vegetarian brown rice sushi, macrobowls, brown rice congee and Kitchari

- Follow instructions on supplements.

If you choose to fast or follow a mono diet, stop eating this diet on day 6 and resume on day 11.

Fasting diet starts day 7-10.

*These foods can be found at your local health food store, alternative grocers or health food section of supermarkets

Other foods allowed:

- raw seeds (chia, hemp, sunflower, sesame, pumpkin, flax)
- walnuts, almonds
- lentils, mung beans, adzuki beans, sprouted soy, miso and tempeh sesame seeds, tahini,
- humus (pure ingredients)
- Nutritional Yeast is an excellent source of vegan protein (plus B vitamins)
- Organic sprouted tofu and tempeh if extra protein is needed.
- Otherwise best to stay away from foods high on food chain. (if necessary: boiled eggs, ocean-going fish, free-range chicken)
- Unsweetened almond, organic soy, hemp, coconut and brown rice milk

Drinking organic vegetable broths is alkalizing as well.

RECIPE: Boil a Yukon gold potato, a carrot, a whole onion, drink the liquid. It catches a lot of magnesium and potassium otherwise lost. It's alkalizing and good for digestion. You can also cook rice or congee in this.

Recipes: Chia Pudding
By Chef James Ray

½ Cup chia seeds
2 C water

1 Cup coconut milk
1 t vanilla extract, vanilla powder OR 1 vanilla bean (scraped)
pinch of salt

1. In a large mixing bowl, pour water over chia seeds and whisk (let sit 5 minutes while you prepare other ingredients, whisk occasionally)
2. Mix coconut milk, vanilla, and salt in separate bowl.
3. Whisk all ingredients together thoroughly and let sit 5 minutes.

While waiting for pudding to set, get some toppings ready.
Coconut slivers, blueberries and cacao nibs are all easy and delicious.
This recipe is so creamy coconut !

THERAPEUTIC CALORIE RESTRICTION:

OPTIONAL FASTING: DAY 7-10: *Studies show that in order your genetic predisposition towards chronic disease such as cancer, Alzheimer's, Diabetes can be reset by fasting, consuming 0 calories and only water and herbal teas for 3 days. There is an optional fast within with cleanse. The most effective fast is to consume 0 calories per day. I have also included the option of a mono diet. NOTE: If you already have a chronic illness such as heart disease or diabetes you may not be able to follow the fast, in which case you continue the brown rice diet detox. Systematically lowering caloric intake to 1200 kcals/day will also reset your genes in the long run. Studies show that therapeutic calorie restrictors who eat all the required nutrients in fewer calories age more slowly and develop less chronic disease.*

Continue through Day 14. This diet can be a very difficult venture if you are not prepared. You must have the food in your cupboards and know where you can eat outside. The more you stick with it, the better you will feel. Try your best and concentrate on what you are able to do, not what you aren't able to.

Most vegan restaurants serve a hearty version of a "macrobowl." This dish is easy to throw together at home! Here's a yum-looking recipe from The Kitchen:

Brown Rice Bowl With lentils and Tahini-Miso Dressing

Ingredients
1 tablespoon wheat-free Tamari soy sauce
1 teaspoon brown rice vinegar
1 clove garlic, grated or crushed
4 ounces beluga lentils (or any style)
1 (6-inch) piece dried wakame seaweed
1/4 cup tahini
1 tablespoon light miso
2 teaspoons lemon juice
2 teaspoons grated ginger
About 1/4 cup warm water
4 cups kale cut into 1/2-inch ribbons
2 cups cooked brown rice

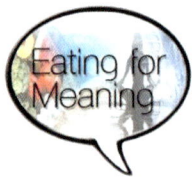

1/2 cup sauerkraut*Most vegan restaurants serve a hearty version of a "macrobowl." This dish is easy to throw together at home! Here's a yummy recipe:

Brown Rice Bowl with Maple-Glazed Tempeh and Tahini-Miso Dressing

Ingredients

1 tablespoon soy sauce

1 tablespoon maple syrup *

1 teaspoon rice vinegar

1 clove garlic, grated or crushed

4 ounces tempeh, cut into 1/4-inch thick slices

1 (6-inch) piece dried wakame seaweed

1/4 cup tahini

1 tablespoon light miso

2 teaspoons lemon juice

2 teaspoons grated ginger

About 1/4 cup warm water

4 cups kale cut into 1/2-inch ribbons

2 cups cooked brown rice

1/2 cup sauerkraut

1 avocado, sliced

1 teaspoon sesame seeds

* Deepen the Detox: To make this recipe even healthier, omit the maple syrup or replace the marinated tempeh with plain organic sprouted tofu. Also, be sure to buy your sauerkraut in the refrigerated section – this is the kind of sauerkraut that contains probiotic live cultures. **Be sure to buy at your local organic grocer or health food store.

Coming off the Detox Diet

It is important to add foods back into your diet gradually. The first reason is that you don't want to shock your system into feeling upset again. The second reason is that this is a perfect opportunity to reintroduce other foods into your diet and observe how they react in your system.

The key point to remember is to introduce only one substance at a time at any given meal. After you have found that a substance is agreeable with you, it may be combined with other foods you are tolerating well

CONTINUE TO DO THE FOLLOWING:
> No canned products.
> Eat raw fruit. Eat fruit by itself: 1/2 before or 2 hours after eating.
> Drink liquids 1/2 hour before or 1 hour after eating for better digestion

YOU MAY CHOOSE TO ADD ANY OF THESE INGREDIENTS IN THE FOLLOWING TIME FRAMES. ONCE YOU FIND THAT YOU TOLERATE THEM WELL YOU MAY CONTINUE TO USE THEM.

➢ *IF you experience a reaction to any foods while coming off the brown rice diet, take 3 days between introductions.*
➢ *It can take up to 10 days for a symptoms of food sensitivity to go away.*

DAY 1-4	bananas			Dairy-free ice-
	cream (e.g. rice dream)			
	organic dried fruit			Wheat free soya
	sauce			
	honey (raw unpasteurized)			Millet
	mushrooms			Amaranth
	tomato sauce (without sugar and preservatives)			Quinoa and
	quinoa pasta			
	avocadoes (great with sandwiches)			Organic Corn, corn
	oil			
	Wheat-free/gluten free bread			Safflower oil
	100% yeast free rye bread			Sunflower oil
	Rice pasta/rice noodles			Organic Canola oil
	Buckwheat/Kasha			Sesame oil
	organic Strawberries			(no hydrogenated
	oils)			
DAY 5-7	Brazil nuts	Pecans	Sesame seeds	
	Almonds			
	Walnuts	Hazelnuts	Tahini spread	Almond
	butter			
				Almond
	milk (unsweetened)			
	(no peanuts, peanut butter, macadamia nus or pistachios)			
DAY 8-10	Salmon	Trout	Sardines	Halibut
	Mackerel	Herring	Cod	White
	fish			
	(no shellfish), if it is necessary to have tuna and salmon from cans use fish			

	canned in water				
DAY 11-14	Chicken	Turkey	Duck	Lamb	
	Eggs				
	(organic meets and free-range eggs are preferred)				
DAY 15-18	Spelt	Lentils	Beans:	lima	pinto
	adzuki				
	barley	Chickpeas		navy	mung
	red				
	oats	Split peas		kidney	white
	black				
	kamut	Black-eyed peas		fava	
	(make sure to soak and rinse your beans, peas before cooking)				
DAY 19-20	Gee	Yogurt	Feta Cheese		
DAY 21	Whole grain products (bread, pasta, baked goods)				
DAY 22	rennet-free whole raw-milk cow cheese (unpasteurized)				

Which foods are not helping you with your health goals?

1.
2.
3.
4.
5.
6.
7.
8.
9.
10

18 EPIGENETICS: PUTTING IT ALL TOGETHER

Exercise 18 and beyond = ***Can you eat like this MOST of the time?***	
<u>**Supplements:**</u>	

If you have gone through this book, you have likely changed your habits and the staples of your diet. You may even find, you want to follow this plan for a while.

DAY	SAMPLE MEAL A	SAMPLE MEAL B
WAKE UP BITTERS AND WARM WATER	Warm water with a squeeze of fresh lemon juice or 1 tsp of apple cider vinegar, shakes of Angostura bitters, aloe juice or 1 inch leaf, 1 cup water additionally. Hydrate and detox in the morning. Take supplements	Warm water with a strong green tea, bitter tea, gentian, dandelion, neem with no milk. 1-2 cups of water additionally. Take supplements
BREAKFAST 7AM	1-2 soft or hard boiled organic eggs, 1 cup fresh fruit and or 1 cup salad with a sprinkle of raw sunflower, pumpkin, hemp or seeds of choice, piece of gluten-free or sprouted bread, or ½ cup quinoa 1 tablespoon raw olive oil, ½ avocado, coconut oil or cultured butter.	½ cup of whole oats oatmeal, gluten-free cereal, plain unsweetened yogurt, 1 cup of fresh fruit salad-berries, apples, pears or lower sugar fruits in your area. 1 glass of unsweetened, almond or rice milk or fresh milk with turmeric.
SNACK 10AM	1 cup of Raw veggies and hummus, gluten-free crackers like *Mary's Gone*, or a handful of raw almonds and an apple or pear. 2 cups water	Rawbar, ProBar Superfood Slam or Superberry and greens OR 1 tablespoon of natural peanut butter with an apple or pear. 2 cups water
LUNCH 12-2PM	2 cups of broccoli or salad greens, beets, carrots, etc. 1 sweet potato or blue/red potato with skin, 4 oz. free range meat, wild fish or 1 cup of rice, pita bread, white potatoes Finish meal with digestive tea or Angostura herbal bitters and water to reduce gas and bloating.	1 cup Lentil or bean salad with mixed vegetables and onion, side salad, bowl of vegetable or soup, 1 cup of quinoa or high fiber pasta/rice noodles. See plate breakdown for portions.
SNACK 4PM	2 handfuls of raw walnuts, seeds, raisins or KIND Plus Walnut Macadamia + Protein with	Smoothie: 1 teaspoon coconut or almond butter, ½ banana or ½

	Peanuts Bar, 2 cups water or an apple or pear dipped in Nutritional Yeast	avocado, ¼ cup of carrot juice, water or unsweetened rice or almond milk 1 cup of water or 2 squares of almond dark chocolate an a ½ cup berries
DINNER 6:30-7PM	2 cups Vegetarian stew or chicken curry, 2 cups of green salad and/or 1 cup cooked greens or carrots. 1 teaspoon raw olive oil and fresh lemon or lime, 1 tablespoon of olive oil, coconut oil or olive oil. 1 cup rice or pasta. Fennel tea or a sipper of alcoholic bitters/digestive or aperitif—Campari, Jaegermeister, etc. Remember portion size	1 cup Miso soup, 2 cups salad or 1 cup cooked greens, 1 cup brown rice, 8 piece salmon sashimi, or 8 rolls. OR 4-6 oz. sirloin, side of steamed or sautéed greens and 1 potato plus 1-2 cups of green mixed salad with balsamic vinaigrette or oil and vinegar dressing or Caesar salad with house-made dressing or , clear broth soup Finish with green, dandelion, chamomile tea or fennel seeds in water to make your own tea Glass of red wine

What foods would you add into to your weekly diet?

_____
_____
_____
_____
_____
_____
_____
_____
_____
_____

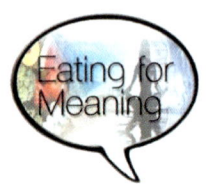

BUT EVENTUALLY YOU MAY FIND YOU CAN EAT WHATEVER

YOU WANT BECAUSE YOU ARE EATING FOR MEANING

❖ Are you willing to change? Willing to change, be exposed to something new, chase a dream, fall down, reach a goal, Mt. Everest. What's your Mt. Everest?

❖ Health is beauty- working on your health, self-healing, self-love, self-care, inside and out, arteries, cells, colon, skin, energy, aura, shining and bright.

❖ Health and beauty come from inside the mind, within the soul. It shines like a light to others who are affected. It's shining to you right now. And it turns your gene expression off and away from aging, obesity, cancer and other chronic disease. Once you understand the connection your food has to the world around you, and the effect this food then has on you, you then have power to change. I am happy to show you a new way.

❖ Do you wish to reprogram your vision of food? Reprogram you, reprogram your metabolism, reprogram your purpose.

❖ Devise a new method of conscious, guilt-free eating, dieting, and nourishing your body under a different mentality.

❖ The powers trying to drag you down:
  o It's harder to change your diet long term than they say because of all the factors against you. Which ones affect you the most? Who do you listen to decide what to eat? Who taught you to eat? Did you listen? Did you rebel? why? It's about YOU now. You can't help others before you help yourself. Children follow what parents do not what parents say. They are smart. They see think
  o Marketing: Big Food as powerful as big tobacco and big pharma. How to avoid falling prey to the vultures, who feed off weaknesses of others. They are out to get your money. Out to win you over to buy their food.
  o Don't believe the hype! The healthiest foods have no packaging. No nutrition labels and only 1 ingredient.

AUTHOR

Millennia (Millie) Lytle, ND, MPH, CNS has a passion for solving health puzzles. Dr. Millie earned a four-year doctorate diploma from the Canadian College of Naturopathic Medicine (2002).

Dr. Millie is a published researcher, radio host and author. Upon moving to New York, she mentored with nutritional biochemistry wizard, Jerry Hickey, pharmacist and nutritionist. She is a licensed ND with the District of Columbia DOH, a licensed nutrition specialist with the BCNS and a member of the NYANP. She is a co-founder of the Association of Perinatal Naturopathic Doctors (APND). She has been published in NDNR, NatPath and is a contributor to NPLEX pharmacology examinations.

Dr. Millie is the Author of Eating for Meaning Workbook, Eating for Meaning Guide to Detox, Guide to Fertility and The Food for Mood Diet; Eat for Your Brain Not Your Stomach. She teaches her nutrition program, Eating for Meaning, at the New York Open Center to help others transform their relationship to food and get to the root-cause-resolution of illness. She practices Naturopathic Medicine in Brooklyn, virtually and at Tournesol Wellness, where she is a member of a primary care team in New York.

Wishing you the best health,

Dr. Millie
Millennia Ruth Lytle, ND, MPH, CNS

www.milliesays.com

Printed in Great Britain
by Amazon.co.uk, Ltd.,
Marston Gate.